THAT'S A WRAP!

THE STEP-BY-STEP GUIDE TO 29 EASY AND ELEGANT
HEAD WRAP STYLES FOR WOMEN IN CHEMOTHERAPY

Lou Gideon

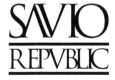

SAVIO
REPVBLIC

A SAVIO REPUBLIC BOOK
An Imprint of Post Hill Press
ISBN: 978-1-68261-825-7

That's a Wrap!
The Step-by-Step Guide to 29 Easy and Elegant Head Wrap Styles
for Women in Chemotherapy
© 2018 by Lou Gideon
All Rights Reserved

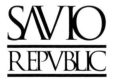

posthillpress.com
New York • Nashville

Published in the United States of America
Printed in China

"…no longer is the promise that bad things can never happen—
rather, the promise is the strength and the faith
to create meaning and beauty from loss."

David J. Wolpe, *Why Faith Matters*

Dedicated to all the loving hearts who helped complete this project,
but most especially, to my dear husband, Walt.

TABLE OF CONTENTS

A SMALL PREVIEW...

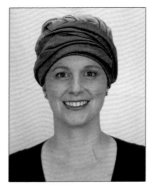
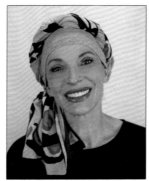
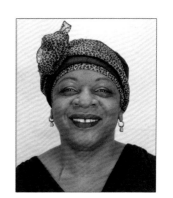
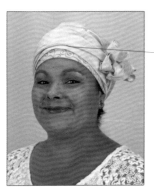
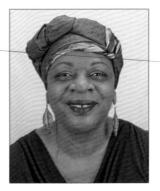
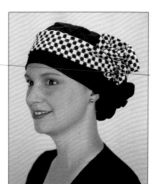
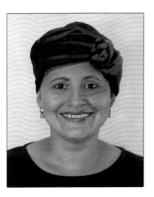
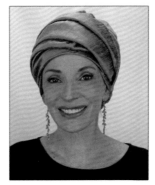
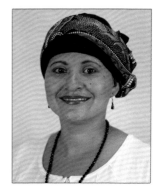

INTRODUCTION: A LETTER FROM LOU

Dear Reader,

When I was diagnosed with breast cancer in March 2009, one of the first things I was concerned about, besides wanting to do everything I could possibly do to beat this awful disease, was how I would cope with losing my hair.

Going into hiding certainly wasn't an option. This malady had surfaced mid-paragraph in a jam-packed chapter of my life, complete with meetings and luncheons and projects and, heck, I even had a party or two on the calendar! Bald? Really? For at least 10 months? Okaaaaayyyyyy...

Both of my medical teams at Duke University Medical Center and Hope Women's Cancer Center in Asheville addressed the situation by providing me with a couple of head-covering catalogues.

Now, even though I found both of these medical establishments to be superb in their overall treatment, I have to admit that, for me, these catalogues just didn't nail it. I even found myself starting to get a little bit depressed, flipping through the pages—not that there weren't some lovely offerings in there that I'm sure would work well for some women, because there truly were. But, when it came to finding something that was my style, it just wasn't happening.

But, a lack of style simpatico with these brochures was only part one of what sent me into the blues.

The part that really pinched my heart, as I looked at all those glossy photos, was the apple-cheeked health of the models. These women weren't bald underneath all those hats, scarves, and wigs—not with fawnlike eyelashes and eyebrows worthy of Brooke Shields! Who did they think they were kidding?

And, even though the gorgeous young things sporting the wigs and wraps were smiling politely, I just couldn't relate to them. In the first place, there was no mention of any of them being cancer survivors themselves, which led me to assume, perhaps incorrectly, that they couldn't possibly relate to what I was facing. God forbid they should ever have to go through such a diagnosis, but you understand my point.

Besides that, can I tell you how ridiculous some of those twenty-something models looked in a few of the more grandma-type styles? It brought to mind the nubile lovelies sporting pastel cotton housecoats in the fashion ads at the back of *The National Enquirer*. You just know that not one of those gals has anything that even faintly resembles such a frock hanging anywhere in her closet! (Hey! I stand in line at the grocery store too!)

Tossing the catalogues aside, I slouched deeper into the comforting fuzziness of my office easy chair. What was I going to do? What other choices did I have, if any? And, whom could I call who might be able to give me those choices?

I realized that what I needed, besides a great head-cover plan, was a personal mentor—to hold the hand of someone who had already been through the bald experience and had successfully come out the other side. I needed a "how-to-look-your-best-while-coping-well-with-losing-your-hair" coach!

Since I couldn't find that coach, I considered the options that were available to me a little further. Right off the bat, I knew that wearing a wig wouldn't work for me. I had tried them before for fun, but every time I put one on, within minutes, my scalp started itching like crazy and I'd feel the pangs of an oncoming headache. Plus, it's a dead giveaway that the hair you're fluffing is not attached to your head when you're sliding a chopstick up the side of your scalp to try to quell an incessant itch.

And, the "Chemo and Cancer Headwraps and Scarves" that I googled online just weren't my style, either. Besides, how would I know if the colors would actually match my wardrobe if I did order something from a catalogue or website?

That got me to thinking. What if I could find a great material myself that would add some bulk to a bald head like hair does, looks great, and feels comfortable? Then I could add accent pieces with color or a print that I chose to that base piece.

I perused the local fabric store, brought home what I thought might be some promising selections of material, and began a series of trial-and-error experimentation for the next few days: wrapping, unwrapping, tying, twisting, tucking, and cutting until I came up with a few looks that I really liked. I began by wearing those simple styles, but I kept playing with the concept throughout my treatment until I eventually found myself wearing lots of different looks that I really liked!

After receiving innumerable "What kind of wonderful hat is that?" and "Where can I get one of those?" questions and compliments, I felt this malleable wrap I was wearing needed a special name. I decided to call it a "Clochellay" (pronounced *klo-shuh-LAY*), because once it's on—no matter which variation of the style you are sporting—it still looks like a combination of the French cloche hat and the African gele wrap. ("Gele" is a Nigerian word for a female head wrap.) And, isn't "Clochellay" a lot more fun than saying "head wrap," "cancer scarf," or "do-rag"?

The Clochellay is an all-encompassing word for a head wrap, usually made with a base of Dupioni silk with an added accent piece that you create to match your wardrobe. It's easy and quick to wrap, feels great on your head, and, with only a few swatches of material or scarves that you already own, you can create a multitude of combinations!

Incidentally, during the months while I was wearing a Clochellay daily, there were a few occasions when someone would comment that, though they loved the look, they were afraid it wouldn't look good on them, or that they wouldn't be able to wrap it.

Whenever that happened, I would take my Clochellay off and show them how to wrap it for themselves. Every single time, the women were delighted by how easy it was to wrap, as well as surprised by how great they looked. The Clochellay styles are flattering to all types of faces!

Whether you're facing your hair loss now or are already without your tresses, it is my hope that, through this book, I can be that person that's there for you, like the coach I had wished for, holding your hand. I write this book to uplift you during the process, give you some information and ideas about how you might approach it, and, finally, to teach you the twenty-nine different styles in which you can wrap that beautiful head of yours!

Love,
Lou

P.S. Incidentally, all models in the following pages were either undergoing chemo or had just finished chemo, with the exception of me. I experienced chemo-related hair loss in 2009.

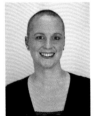 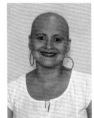 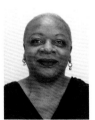 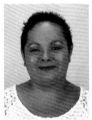 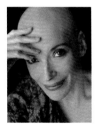

Our team of head wrap models are: Kristin, Yvette, Theresa, Maria, and me.

CHAPTER 1: MY HAIR'S GOING *WHERE?*

February 28, 2009

It was a late Friday afternoon, and I had just arrived home from a weeklong business trip to Florida. My unpacked bags remained in the entryway, holding memories from the past seven days that I wanted to share with my family, as well as my unshareable dirty laundry. I was standing in the kitchen, making tea and laughing about something with my fiancé, Walt, when I summoned the courage to ask if he had heard back from the doctor's office regarding the recent breast biopsy I had undergone. I had requested they contact him with the report instead of me, as I didn't want to worry about it while I was away on business.

"Okay. Did the doctor call?" I asked, still chuckling from Walt's remark, whatever it was.

His eyes glazed a bit. "Uh…yeah. They did." His lips pressed together to form the kind of smile that carries a deep sigh with it.

My body went ice cold and time jerked to a stop. "I have cancer."

Walt, true to form, immediately launched into trying to make me feel better. "Well, yes, but the doctor said that it's the size of a grain of salt and that they should easily be able to remove it with a lumpectomy."

A grain of salt? Lumpectomy? *Well, that's not absolutely horrible,* I told myself. *It might even be good, in fact, if you have to receive a cancer diagnosis. At least they feel they can take care of it.*

Still, I began toppling fear-first into a long, deep abyss.

Walt continued, "We have an appointment this coming Tuesday to talk with your doctor and schedule the lumpectomy."

Okay. Okay. Well, we'll find out what they have to say further on Tuesday, then.

He wrapped his arms around me, and the silence that enveloped us said everything. We were in this together.

Moments later, we went downstairs to my mom's apartment on the lower level of our house to try to enjoy the "welcome home meal" she had prepared for my return. Looking back, I did a fairly good job that evening of pushing the cancer diagnosis out of my mind, at least enough to tell stories from my previous week during dinner. But when I sprinkled a bit of salt onto my vegetables, I found myself fixated on the individual grains as they melted away into the food.

In the week that followed, however, we learned that the "grain" turned out to be more like a couple of the larger, clumpy bits you find in saltshakers near the ocean. There were two tumors: one around three centimeters in size, and the other "surprise" tumor close to five centimeters. Seems my dense breasts resembled the moors on a foggy night in England when it came to trying to see what might be hiding behind every corner, just waiting to attack.

I proceeded with the lumpectomy, which was followed by that ever-so-festive period of waiting for the results. The phone call brought more lovely news: The lab report revealed that the surgery had left unclean margins on three sides, and that the cancer was present in two out of three sentinel lymph nodes.

It now had a name: Stage IIB invasive ductal carcinoma.

Chemotherapy, radiation, and a bilateral mastectomy now loomed on my calendar in bright red letters, promising a date with the "Anti-Fun." No last-minute cancellations allowed. The thought of "Why me?" never crossed my mind, but I must admit that I did wonder, "How did this happen?" as I had no history of cancer in my family, strove to eat a healthy diet, was a very positive person, exercised regularly, and never smoked.

I quickly learned that there would be no answer forthcoming. Nobody can tell you how you develop cancer, or why you get it, but the angry woman who lives down the street who eats nothing but sugar and fried pork seems to be the picture of health. There's no crystal ball in which you can see if you are going to "make it," or for how long you'll live.

I found these unanswered questions had me feeling somewhat akin to what a person might experience after watching a sci-fi thriller whose ending was left open for interpretation. That, multiplied by a thousand.

I wanted someone to come out of the sky, point a god-like finger in my direction, and say, "If you follow these procedures and do exactly what so-and-so says and eat *this* way for the rest of your life, you'll live to be 107 and die in your sleep of a heart attack."

Oh, how I wanted someone to be able to tell me that!

But then, I realized that the answers to such questions had never been there. Ever. I never had a definite life-expectancy guarantee prior to my cancer diagnosis. And further, such guarantees don't exist for *anybody*.

Having swallowed this reality pill, I sat down to try to figure out what other substances I could look forward to swallowing or having injected in the upcoming months. I picked up the Cancer Care notebook I'd been given and began reviewing the treatment dance card my oncologist had given me. What was I facing, really?

The notebook was formidable, to say the least. Its three-ring binder had a 2 ½-inch circumference, if that tells you anything, and it was filled with page upon page of information containing pharmaceutical names and procedures with which I wasn't exactly familiar. Botox, I knew. Promethazine or dexamethasone, not so much. I decided to break down the highlights to try to make each one sit more comfortably in my psyche:

- Six rounds of chemo—with each one to be administered at three-week intervals. That meant I'd be cocktailing from May to August. Well, I always felt that summers passed the most quickly of all the seasons, so maybe this little belief of mine would help the days seem to go faster while I wasn't exactly feeling my best. (Good! I liked that. This idea sounded somewhat convincing, right?)

- Then there were three surgeries looming. A bilateral mastectomy, followed by the insertion of expanders to stretch my breast skin, and, after that was completed, implants. I could handle that. I had lived for twenty years in Los Angeles, for goodness sakes—"Land of the Fake Boobs by Choice"—and was accustomed to being around surgically enhanced breasts. And, though I never would have chosen to augment mine for looks, if safer models were a necessity for my health, I figured I might as well embrace the concept.

- Radiation, I didn't have to deal with yet, and, perhaps, I wouldn't have to at all. Whether I qualified for that particular treatment was totally dependent upon what they found in my tissue post-mastectomy. And, since I refused to concern myself over something that might not even happen, I temporarily filed radiation away into a mental cubby—to be opened later, if ever.

So far so good, I thought. I've manipulated almost everything that I'm facing into a neat little can-do cubicle inside my head.

My head. Oh. There still remained the matter of how to handle my soon-to-be bald head.

On a good note, I knew that being bald around my house held no worries. Oh, the dogs might cock their heads at me for a day or two, the way they do at each

15

other when one of them gets a particularly close-shaven puppy cut. But in the end, they wouldn't give a Greenie what I looked like as long as I remembered when it was their dinnertime. As for my sweet mom and Walt—they didn't care what I looked like as long as I was on the road to recovery.

But, what about business meetings? Dining out with friends? That upcoming fancy shindig Walt and I were expected to attend?

It had been suggested to me, more than once, that perhaps a wig might be in order. But, I found wigs to be scratchy and uncomfortable when I wore them in plays or on Halloween. The thought of donning one every single time I stepped outside for the next few months made me feel like a reluctant drag queen. I wanted to look good, but I wanted it without suffering the angst that came along with it.

That being said, I was still in need of a solution enough to pry my mind open and do a little research online. There, I learned that wigs range in price from around $99 to over $5,000, depending on the quality. I also learned that we have several wig stores here in Asheville. So, I chose the closest one, called my girlfriend Janie to go with me, and we took a drive across town.

This particular salon turned out to be a delightful place run by a charmingly eccentric British woman. A wig wearer herself, she had a genuine enthusiasm for fake hair that gave me the much-needed confidence that suggested I would be safe and taken care of in her presence. Even my ever-protective Janie gave the salon and owner a thumbs-up as we were perusing her selections. After I had selected a few style possibilities, I was ushered to her fitting station, where she began coaxing my tendrils into submission and eventually secured the mass of tight curls underneath a head stocking. The moment had arrived. I lifted my favorite wig-choice off its display head and, as Janie watched, the British wig-shop owner and I started pulling it into place.

Thirty minutes later, I found myself being stared at by a table full of unhappy-looking styrofoam head rejects, my scalp itched like crazy, and I was fighting an oncoming headache. No matter how well-intended the British owner or how vast her wig selection, I had to unhappily accept the fact that wearing a wig just wasn't going to be an option for me. I politely begged off, though I must admit I *did* enjoy her complimentary wine and being a redhead for a few short moments.

So, the question as to what I was going to do with my head remained.

I went to my closet and dug into the wonderful collection of scarves that my friends had begun sending once the news of my diagnosis was out. There were so many beautiful patterns and textures, surely one or two would work? Unfortunately, the sizes weren't quite right. Though they might look great around my neck or shoulders, I just couldn't seem to get any of them to look right as a head covering.

The smallest of them shouted "do-rag." This look is not exactly me. Walt owns a motorcycle—it's practically a prerequisite for living in these beautiful mountains—and I know that riding has its merits for some people. Still, I don't want to look like I just jumped off the rear end of a Harley.

Midsized scarves might look passable in the front, but they left a portion of my scalp peeking out in the back, which I equated to wearing a crop-top over the age of thirty. No matter how many stomach crunches I might do on a daily basis, there were certain portions of my body that I just didn't want showing in public at this point in my life.

And, though the largest scarves might have provided total coverage, they still gave me a domed-look, which I feel would announce "cancer victim" everywhere I might go.

I thought back to the catalogues that my medical teams had given me. Nothing there was going to work, because, as I mentioned, the styles didn't really fit my taste. Along with that, it didn't help that the choices made in their carefree-looking models ticked me off in that none of them looked like they could ever relate to waking up the morning after a chemo-session with their energy flat-lined, their fingernails coming loose, and 32 ulcers on their tongue. (Yep. I counted 32 ulcers after my first chemo.)

And, I hope they never do.

Always up for ideas, however, I googled "head wraps for hair loss," where I found a wide selection of various fashions ranging in price from $10 to $40. Now, truth be told, I thought that a few of them were reminiscent of someone named Hattie Mae whiling away an afternoon churning butter. Others definitely showed some promise design-wise, but the prints weren't my cup of tea. And, even if I found one or two for which I liked both the design and the print, how could I be sure that the brown shade on my computer screen would actually match the brown in my favorite suit? Not to mention the blue? (You *know* how difficult matching blues can be!) Besides that, many of the materials looked fuzzy. "Fuzzy" wasn't a fashion statement I wanted to make—bald or not.

Then it occurred to me that even if I had found several head wraps that I liked, wouldn't I get tired of wearing the same ones for nine months?

Yes! I would!

At least I was learning what I felt I was really looking for from all of this. It was a head wrap that was comfortable to wear for hours, looked great on me, would perfectly match my wardrobe, and that I could vary, style-wise.

Something...*other* than what I was finding in the catalogues or online.

A few days later, I was still brooding over all of this when I found myself driving past a local fabric store on the way home from the dry cleaners. I used to love to tie things into my hair to give it fullness during the years I lived in Los Angeles. Maybe I could figure something out that would work for me now.

I walked in, feeling a little gloomy as my first chemo treatment was scheduled for the following Tuesday and I knew that time for a solution was rapidly drawing to a close. Looking for inspiration, I began strolling through the fabric aisles. Past the flannel plaids that would only add ruggedness to a bald gal. Past the festive calicos, the creamy chenille's, the Day-Glo rayons that begged to adorn a bastion of baton twirlers.

And then I saw it, lined up on a shelf near the back corner. An old friend.

Dupioni silk.

Years ago, when I was travelling in the Far East as a nightclub singer, I learned the many pleasures of Dupioni, or "Thai" silk. It's not only gorgeous—rich looking with an elegantly understated shimmer—but it can also *do anything*.

Its texture is such that it looks even better wrinkled, like an expensive linen, only finer. It stays in place well and has enough chutzpah in its silken fibers to hold some shape, an excellent perk when you're going to be dealing with a domed head for a little while.

I excitedly went out to the car to pull a few pieces of plastic-sheathed clothing from the dry cleaning I had just picked up, then went back inside and pulled down a couple of luscious brown bolts.

One matched my brown suit perfectly.

"Can you cut this for me about, oh, yea-and-a-half long?" I held out my arms at the cutting station to show the clerk approximately how much I wanted. "I made a B minus in seventh grade home economics class. I'm afraid I'm not much of a seamstress..."

She smiled, pulled the measuring tape from my left fingers to my right to measure the length I was demonstrating, then added the half-length, cut, folded, and handed me the cloth, along with a price slip she'd written.

"What are you going to do with it, then?" she asked.

"I'm not quite sure. I'll let you know in a minute."

I ducked into the ladies' room and began fooling around with the material, realizing very quickly that I was going to need another foot or so in length if I wanted it to go around my head twice with some left over for tying. And, it was way too bulky. The bolts came in 44-inch widths, so I'd also need it cut in half length-wise to make it work.

I returned to the cutting counter.

My junior high sewing teacher would have been proud, because, this time, instead of holding my arms out to get somewhere near the amount I now wanted, I asked the clerk to help me measure my head, which turned out to be 22 inches around. I figured that I should double that amount so it could wrap twice and leave enough material to tie and secure it in place. We decided that 13 extra inches would do it, so, this time, she cut 57 inches for me. I also had her cut it length-wise down the middle to reduce the bulk.

When I got back to the ladies' room and tried again—presto! It wrapped, tucked, and looked great! I walked out to the cutting table, head wrap in place.

I lifted my hands towards my head. "What do you think?"

"I like it! Are you going to a party or something?" the clerk asked.

"Kind of. At least, I know they'll be serving cocktails." I smiled.

I went back to the Dupioni silks and pulled out a beautiful cream bolt, as well as a black. I had them cut for my head measurement as before, as well as cut down the center length-wise to take out the bulk again. That gave me two head wraps in each color. So, not counting the first one that I had her cut too short, I now had six wraps (in three colors) for $75.95.

Next, I knew that I needed some accent pieces. As the spring began to return to my step—as it always does when you're having fun—I made my way around the store in search of materials that would work well with the brown, black, and cream Dupioni silk I had just chosen. I thought about my summer/fall wardrobe, as my bald months were going to be at the minimum June through November, and began pulling out other bolts. I could choose any material for the accents: cotton, linen, silk, flimsy see-through, whatever. These fabrics didn't need to have substance to them, because I'd already gotten that with my Dupioni base material. This time, I could choose for colors and patterns alone.

It was a lot less expensive to purchase the accent material because I only needed a small amount of fabric, enough to fold into thirds (so the edges wouldn't fray when I wore it), then wrap once around my head, leaving a little left over to create a decorative "knot" of some kind, or to hang down, if I wanted. Since the bolts came in 44-inch widths, I knew that 44 inches would be enough material to accomplish this with plenty of extra left over. So, I used the 44 inches as my "length." I then had the clerk cut them at 12 inches for width. (Remember, I was going to fold it into thirds, so the final accent strip of fabric would be about 4 inches wide.)

I chose 21 different accent pieces ranging in price from $3.99 to $9.99 per yard. My cost came to around $56.

Keep in mind that accent pieces made of solid color Dupioni look great, as well. Even though materials with prints are compelling, they won't always go as easily with your wardrobe. So, make sure that you get a few pieces of solid accent colors in Dupioni, as well as in other fabrics to mix and match for when you are wearing clothes with a pattern.

And, as for that B minus I'd received in seventh-grade sewing class, I found a non-sewing solution to any hemming I might face by purchasing two packages of iron-on hem tape, which were $1.65 apiece.

One hour and approximately $142 after entering the fabric store, I left with enough material to create 63 different looks, which I would accomplished by tying one of the accent colors onto each of the three base wraps. But, I could achieve 63 *more* different looks if I used the accent colors *under* the base wraps (which I'll show you how to do in this book), and three more looks if I wanted to combine the base wraps themselves.

That added up to 132 days, or almost 4 ½ months of different looks! And, this wasn't even taking into consideration those wonderful scarves I had at home that could work as base and accent pieces as well!

Now, I was getting somewhere. (Later, when I went home and got really creative, I realized that the different possibilities with what I had purchased at the fabric store alone were actually closer to 200. But, again, I'll show you how to achieve that later in this book.)

By the time I pulled out of my parking space, my depressed mood had lifted, replaced by a tinge of excitement. If I had to be bald, I wanted to feel the best I could about it. I felt I'd found my answer as to how to do it, and it only cost around $142. One wig would have cost me at least that much! And, the head wraps were so much softer and more comfortable than a wig.

Now that my spirits were up, I decided not to wait to let my hair fall out bit by bit. How depressing would *that* be—trying to hold onto something that's definitely on its way out?

I went home and began planning a "hair shedding party."

CHAPTER 2: LET'S HAVE A PARTY!

Like most women, I consider my hair to be a big part of my "look." The idea of losing it was scary. De-feminizing. Threatening.

Let's face it. I was absolutely horrified.

Since I knew that it would begin falling out approximately four weeks after my first chemo treatment, I decided not to wait for the awful day when I would run my fingers through my hair and have a handful in my palm.

I had watched the heartbreaking Farrah Fawcett documentary about her courageous cancer journey, and I had a lump in my throat when I watched Mela Murphy, her dear friend and hairdresser of 18 years, trying to hide Farrah's golden tresses in her pockets as they started to fall out. Mela happened to be my hairdresser, too, for many of the years I had lived in Los Angeles. I adored her.

To tell you the kind of big heart Mela has—I once had a pet squirrel that I had saved from a hovering owl when it was a baby. Its mother had been run over, and when I raised it to be big enough to survive on its own, Mela located a wildlife retreat specially created for such creatures and drove it there to be released into blissful adult squirreldom. You gotta love her.

But, back to the situation at hand. A better alternative to balding slowly, I thought, would be to hold a "Hair Shedding Party," complete with close friends, good wine, and a sharp pair of scissors.

We held it at my house, about a week before my first chemo treatment was scheduled. I wanted to get used to the idea of losing my hair by doing it in a series of steps, each of which I controlled—not the chemo. I asked everybody to please bring a handwritten affirmation for me that I would paste into a beautiful little book and read daily as I was going through my treatment.

The plan was that everyone would take a turn reading their affirmation to me and then cut a piece of my hair, leaving it at about two inches in length. Looking back, it was a real stroke of luck that my friend Janie knew something about cutting hair, and I suggest that you invite someone who knows a little bit about cutting hair, if possible. You'll want someone to be able to shape it after everyone else is finished.

The evening of the gathering, we spent an hour or so visiting, and enjoying our noshes and libations before heading into the kitchen for the main event. Walt kept upbeat music playing in the background; we draped a towel over my shoulders and began the reading and clipping.

Note: You don't want to be in front of a mirror for this. It's a lot more relaxing for the person getting their hair cut if they don't see what's happening *as its happening.* That way, you can focus on the affirmations and love coming from your friends.

What I had secretly feared might be a bit of a sad evening for me turned out to be one of the most festive parties I had ever given, and my private plan to keep up a stiff upper lip gave way to a genuine smile from the heart.

All right...back to the hair-shedding story. The morning after the party, I decided it would be fun to go out to the farmer's market to buy summer plants for my deck-garden. In the middle of filling our cart with herbs, roses, and different, colorful varieties of coleus, the wind whipped up, promising a spring shower. My dear friend Micaela, who was used to having short hair, just kept right on picking out plants.

I, on the other hand, instinctively whipped my hand up to my face to keep my hair from blowing into my eyes and getting plastered to my lip gloss. You women out there with long locks know what I'm talking about! But, my hand only found my cheek...as there was no hair flailing about to protect myself from. How liberating! I dropped my hand back down to the plants in front of me and continued choosing the type of basil I wanted to plant. I wasn't the least bothered by the strong breeze.

A few weeks later, when my hair began to get brittle and little bits were beginning to come loose, it was finally time to buzz my head. And, you know what? Becoming bald was no big deal. In fact, it felt pretty great! Think about it: If you've got to lose your hair for a little while, here's a chance to experience a part of your own body as you've never experienced it before. Running my hand over the top of my head felt wild. And, talk about a timesaver! Not having to deal with my hair added at least three extra hours to my week, at the very least. It also saved me a bundle on the hairdresser and gave me a lot more counter space on my dressing table.

So, who knows how you'll feel once you're bald? By the time your hair begins growing back in, you may have a very different opinion about the whole experience than you did at first. Here's a quick story:

I have a friend in New York, an executive in the entertainment industry, who was diagnosed with breast cancer a few months after I was. Now, this woman had a truly spectacular head of hair. Really gorgeous. She purchased one of those $5,000-ish wigs that looked just like her hair had looked.

She told her friends that she would never go around without that wig until her hair grew out. At first, she couldn't even look at herself in the mirror without it.

Jump ahead six months. She's at a health retreat for a couple of weeks. Being bald has now become a little more comfortable for her, and she decided to take her wig off in the privacy of her room and look in the mirror. Something's changed— she likes what she sees. Then she decides to take the bald look outside.

People are shocked, yes. They thought the hair was hers. But, here was another shock—they can't believe how beautiful she is without her hair.

After the health retreat, she goes back to New York, wearing her wig, but she feels a lot more relaxed about the fact that she's bald underneath it. She meets a wonderful man, and after a few dates, shows him how she looks without the wig. He doesn't care—he's in love with her. Who would have thought this period in her life would be the time when she'd find such a great guy?

So, welcome to the Temporarily Bald Club, which not only can be full of surprises, but also holds a membership larger than you could ever imagine. And, one day, when your hair has all grown back in, you'll find yourself encouraging some other woman who's facing her own hair-loss experience.

CHAPTER 3: GETTING STARTED

If you're like me, you work best from a set of detailed, easy-to-understand instructions. And, that's what I've provided here—step-by-step text supported by plenty of photographs. But, please don't be put off by the number of designs I'm going to give you. In only a few pages, you'll master the basic wrap. It's quite simple once you understand how to do it. And, once you understand that, the rest will be easy! There are only two things to remember:

- The key to a comfortable and beautiful base wrap is Dupioni silk (also known as Thai silk).

- There are two pieces to a basic Clochellay: The *base* wrap and the *accent* wrap.

> **Tip**: When it comes to choosing your base wrap, pick out one or two solid colors that will complement most of your wardrobe. This is where the Clochellay has a big advantage over ordering a head wrap online—you get to test the color-match! Black, brown, blue-jean blue, cream, or white are almost always good choices. I suggest that you take a few pieces of your clothing into the fabric store to make sure that the color tones go well together. A cool-toned brown Dupioni isn't going to look good with that warm-toned brown of your favorite suit. So, take the time to carry the bolts of fabric you've chosen and your wardrobe pieces over to a window to compare them in the sunlight to ensure you get a great match!

HOW TO CALCULATE THE LENGTH OF MATERIAL NEEDED FOR THE CLOCHELLAY BASE WRAP

- Measure the circumference of your head, placing the tape measure just above your ears.

- Double that number.

- Add 14 inches and you've got your personal Clochellay base wrap measurement. You may trim this down a bit once you arrive home, but we'll get to that.

- Keeping your personal Clochellay base wrap measurement number in mind, ask the clerk to cut the bolt of material you have chosen at the closest measurement they can to your number. (Fabric stores will only cut material in certain increments, and of a yard is their smallest increment.)

- Now, we want to cut that piece of material to the proper width. Bolts usually come in 44-inch widths. This is fortunate for anyone making a Clochellay, because the universal width needed for *any* head is 22 inches. So, with bolts being 44 inches wide, this means that you'll get *two* base-wraps out of each piece of material you have them cut!

- Ask the clerk to cut it once more, this time in half *length-wise*. By the way, I always have the clerk cut it instead of waiting to cut it myself when I get home. Fabric store scissors are likely to be a lot sharper than yours, and chances are you'll get a much smoother cut this way.

  Tip: Choose a couple of packages of iron-on hem tape—one tape in the color of your base wrap and another in a hem tape that becomes transparent when ironed. We'll talk about how to use the hem tape a bit later. For now, let's move on to how to choose and measure your accent wraps. The accent wrap is where the real fun begins!

  Tip: When it comes to accent wraps, you can choose material for color and pattern alone, as you'll already have a base wrap providing plenty of texture and shape to your head with the Dupioni. So, be creative and pick out some great materials that will complement your wardrobe! (You can also use scarves you already own, but for now, we'll talk about accent wraps from bolts of material.)

HOW TO CREATE THE CLOCHELLAY ACCENT WRAP

- Ask the clerk to cut the 44-inch wide material you've chosen for your accent wrap to 12 inches in width. That will give you an accent wrap of 44 inches in *length* and 12 inches in *width*. Accent wraps only need a small amount of fabric. The 44-inch length gives you plenty of material to wrap around your head once and still have enough left over to tie it or to secure it in one of the many ways I'm going to show you in this book.

- When you get home, fold the accent piece into thirds or fourths, depending on how wide you want your accent piece to be. Thirds will give you a 4-inch width and fourths will give you a 3-inch width. In my opinion, larger heads look better with wider accent wraps and smaller heads look better with thinner accent wraps. But, test it yourself to see what you like. Since you're only folding, you always have the option to go thinner or wider.

- There's no need to sew the 44-inch length, as the folded edges take care of hiding any loose threads. But, you *will* want to hem tape the 12-inch ends with the transparent iron-on hem tape. This will give the ends a nice stiffness that we'll be using in some of the designs, as well as making sure there's no fraying.

Just FYI, I went a little crazy and chose a *lot* of different accent pieces ranging in price from $3.99 to $21.98 per yard. But remember, I was only purchasing one-third of a yard (12 inches) each time. As a result, my cost for all this wonderful color came to about $56. But you can get by with much less and still have a multitude of options!

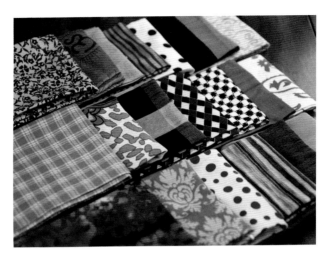

Keep in mind that accent pieces made of solid color Dupioni look great, as well. Even though materials with prints are compelling, they won't always go as easily with your wardrobe. So, make sure that you get a few pieces of solid accent colors in Dupioni, as well as in other fabrics to mix and match when you are wearing clothes with a pattern.

Okay—so let's learn how to wrap! And remember: once you get this base wrap down—and you will within a few attempts—the rest of the designs are going to be a snap, because they all build around this base wrap!

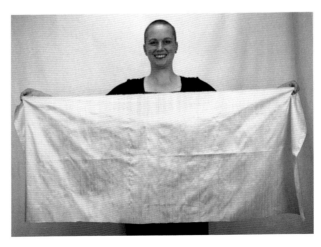

This white piece of Dupioni is 22 inches x 58 inches.

(By the way, from here on out, I'll be using the proper way to state measurements so you'll never get confused: width first, then length.)

Remember I told you in Chapter 1 that the fabric store will require you to round up your Clochellay base wrap measurement to the next highest of a yard? And, that that meant my 58-inch base wrap measurement was rounded off to 60 inches?

Well, because that was 2 inches too much, I needed to trim off the excess before I ironed on the hem tape. You see, if your base wrap is too long, the ends will be floppy on some of the designs—but if it's too short, you won't be able to tuck the ends in when you want to. This is why you'll want to trim your fabric down to the exact length you originally calculated.

Once you've done that, fold each end back about ½ to ¾ inch and iron on the hem tape. This should make your base wrap approximately 1 to 1 ½ inches shorter than your original base wrap number. That's perfect, and you'll begin to understand why in a few more pages.

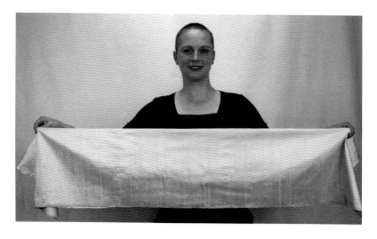

Now you're going to fold the entire piece of material over once, *lengthwise*, and then iron it all the way down the length of the fold so you have a crisp, clean edge.

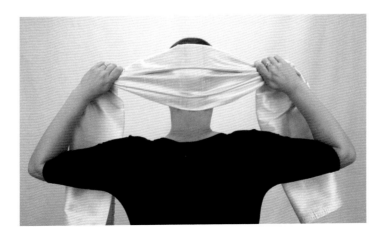

At this point you'll take the folded material and place it at the back of your head, making sure that the *folded side is at the nape of your neck* and the *open side is near the top of your head*, up by the crown. *This is very important!*

Gather the material in your hands so that the top of the fabric doesn't stick up above your crown, but rather, rests just at the top of the back of your head.

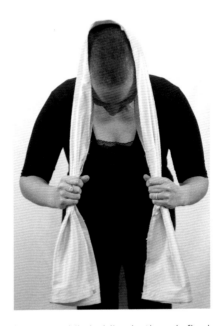

Lean over while holding both ends firmly.

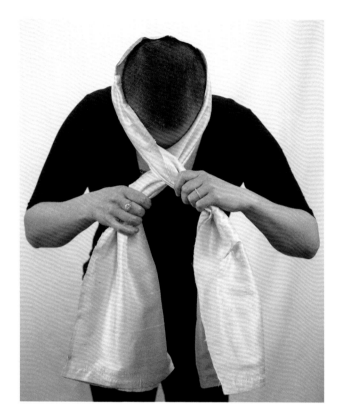

Next, you're going to cross the material over itself in front...placing one of the pieces you are holding in your hands flat across your forehead while allowing the other piece to cross behind it. However, before you attempt to do this, I want you to look at yourself in the mirror and repeat after me: *This next part is a bit tricky, but I promise not to become impatient with myself or anxious about it, as I know I'll soon get it right and be wrapping like a pro!*

Did you say that to yourself? Did you **mean** it?

Good!

What helps me with this step is focusing first on the piece that I'm placing flat against my forehead. I make sure that it's at least semi-smooth, and I try to place it about an inch above my eyebrows, while crossing the other piece of material a bit higher and behind it. (You *will* get the knack of this. It just takes a few attempts until you understand the *feel* of it.) Try not to cross them over at the center, as this gives a "pointy" look at your forehead.

31

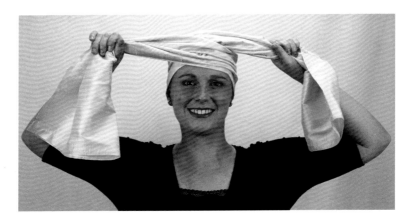

Here's the front view, mid-cross. See how the model has one of the pieces of material wrapped flat across her forehead, with the other one behind it? And, how it's about an inch above her eyebrows? One other thing to be aware of is to try to wrap the material so it leaves the bottom portion of your ears exposed.

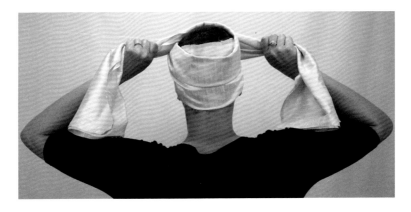

But no worries if the material is covering all of your ears or the outer edges of your eyebrows at this point. You can always push the material higher up your ears and/ or forehead once you get it secured in the back. Here's what it should look like in the back.

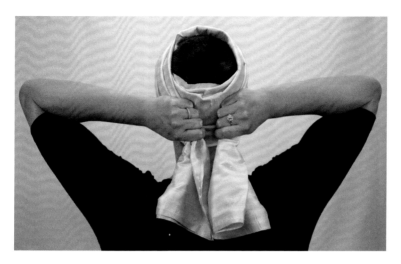

Now you can bring the ends together and begin tying it in the back. Only one crossover is necessary.

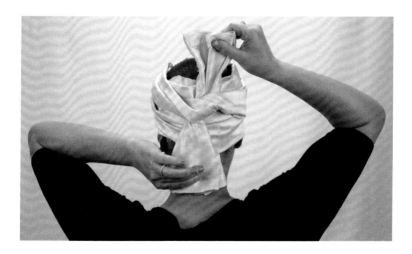

Pull it so it's snugly in place. We'll deal with the ends in a moment.

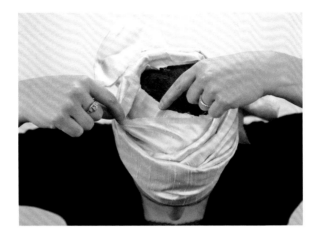

Now you're going to cover the top of your head. Remember how I asked you to keep the folded edge of the material at the nape of your neck, with the two open edges at your crown? This next step is why I said that.

Grab the inside piece (the one resting against the side of your head) of the two open edges firmly with your fingers. It doesn't matter whether you choose the right or left side of your head to do this, as long as you find the innermost piece of material.

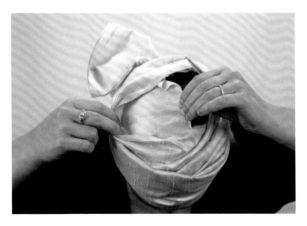

You may have to feel around a little bit to find this piece, but it's there! Next, we're going to gently tug that piece of fabric closest to your scalp across your crown while holding the other, wrapped material at the side of your head firmly in place. The photo shows you exactly what to do. Keep giving the inside piece of material gentle little tugs until it fully covers your crown with a teensy bit extra so you can tuck it into the other side.

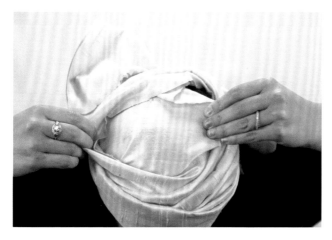

Pull from the point on your head, located directly above your ear, as the model is doing in the photo. If you pull it from near the front of your head, it will pull the portion that you have already wrapped at your forehead out of shape. Tug it until it's all the way across your crown.

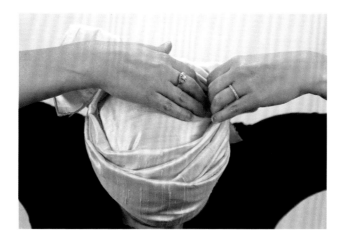

Once you tug it all the way across your crown, tuck the piece that you've just pulled across underneath the other open ends of material on the opposite side of your head.

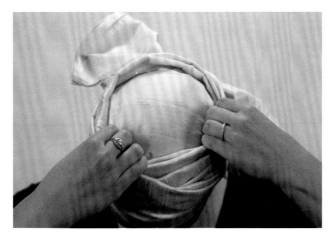

Keep working with it until it's neatly tucked in. Make sure that your crown is completely covered and the folds look finished and intentional, like a hat. Sometimes the top of the Clochellay will look very precise, like it looks on our models, and sometimes it will look more gently rounded. No matter—what's important here is that you get it to cover the top of your head and then tuck it in. You can also tuck in the top edges of the Clochellay just to make it look a little neater, if you like. Our model is doing it here, but it's not absolutely necessary.

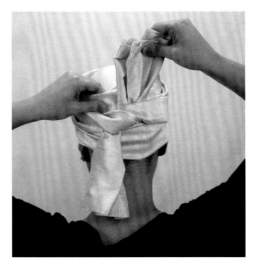

Now that you've covered the top of your head, let's go back to those loose ends you just tied once in the back. Take the top of the back "tie" and tuck it into the material at the top.

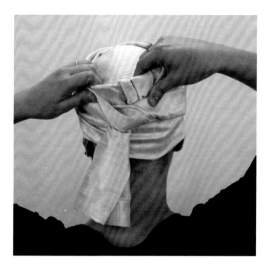

You've got several folds to choose from, so if it won't reach to the top (but hopefully, if you measured correctly at the beginning, you should have enough to reach to the top), just tuck it into itself *somewhere*. This isn't a hard and fast science. Just go for it! Now, take the bottom end of the two ties and tuck it underneath the fold of material at the nape of your neck. Like this!

Voila! No safety pins needed!

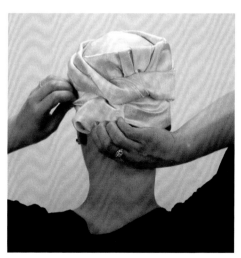 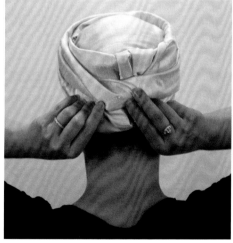

Now that it's in place, you can tug it down a bit to cover what would be your back hairline.

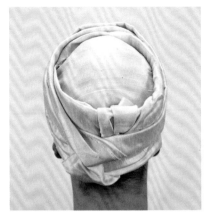

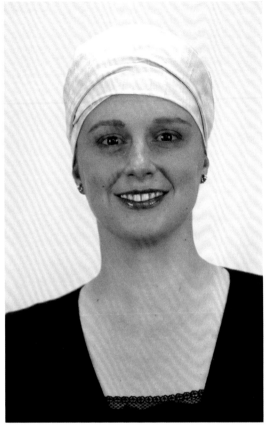

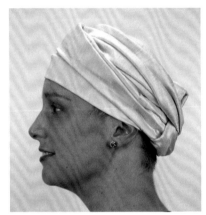

Here's how your Clochellay will appear from the back. And, here's what it should look like, basically, from the side and then the front.

At this point, I always play with it a little near the face, smoothing it across the forehead, making sure that it's about an inch or more above the eyebrows and that it's not too low on the ears, but still covers the upper-tips, and so forth. You'll be surprised how well the material will conform and still hold its shape!

Now for the accent wrap.

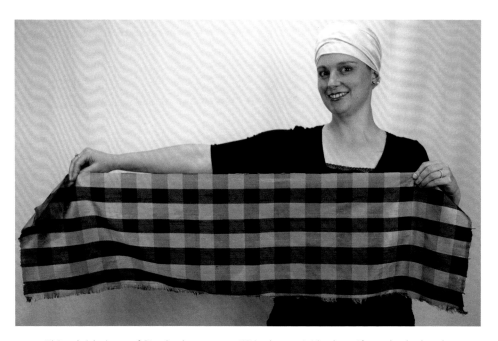

This plaid piece of Dupioni measures 12 inches x 44 inches. If you look closely, you can see that this particular piece is not hemmed. You can hem the ends of your accent pieces with hem-tape, if you like, but unless you're going to be making it into a little *bouffe* (i.e., bouffant-like), or you really like the added stiffness it gives, it's not mandatory.

Now you're going to fold the accent piece either into thirds, fourths, or even fifths—depending on how thick you want your accent piece to be. Make sure there are no shreds of silk fibers dangling.

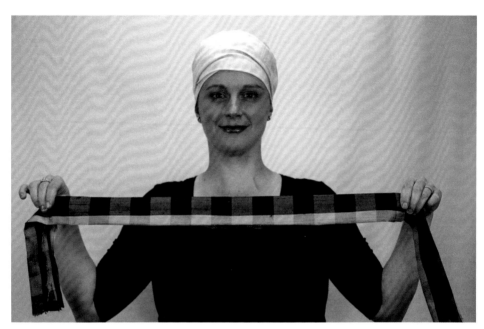

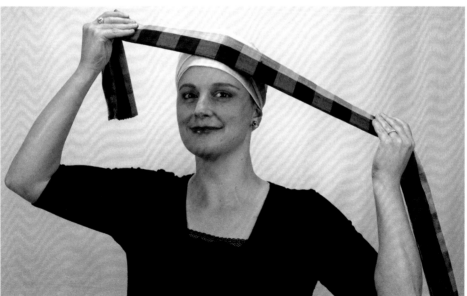

Take hold of it with each hand...and place the center of the accent material at one side of your head.

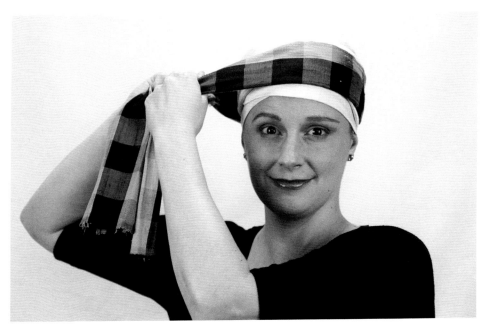

Then pull the ends to the other side so you can tie them above your ear. Tie one end over the other to secure it.

By the way, I don't blame you if you're thinking, "Sheesh! How detailed does she need to be here?" But I figure that "more" is better than "less," just in case. And besides, this first step-by-step chapter is the most comprehensive. After this, we're going to begin doing variations.

So let's keep going!

DESIGN #1

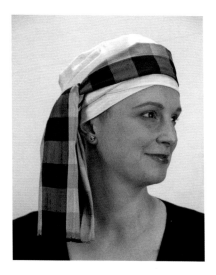

As I'd mentioned, if you want to let the ends dangle, you can hem them with a hem tape that matches the fabric. I hadn't hemmed the edges here, but you get the idea. And, you can leave it only tied once at the side of your head, or you can make it a square knot—whichever you feel stays put the best with the fabric you're using.

DESIGN #2

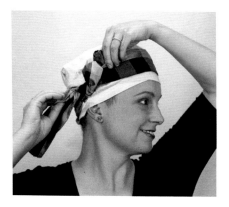

If you decide to tuck it in, take the front part of the "tie" and stuff it into the top of the accent band. There is no hard and fast science here—you can push the fabric into the band any way you like.

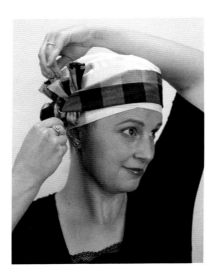

Mine stuck out a bit more than I liked at the bottom, so, to shorten the accent band a bit, I wrapped the "tie" once around the band and then pushed it up under it again. Then I tucked the other portion of the tie underneath the accent band and then pulled it out again to form an "S" shape.

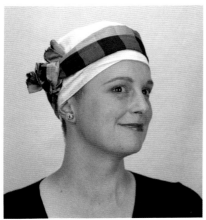 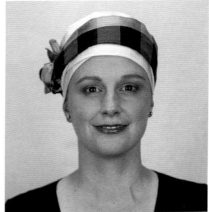

Just play with it a little bit until you get it where you want it. There is no hard and fast rule here! This is it from the side and from the front.

Well done!

So, now you've wrapped your Clochellay and you're out and about town, living your life. But let's imagine that for some reason, you need to take it off for a moment. Here's where a convenient little aspect of the Clochellay comes in. When you need to remove it in the middle of the day, you should be able to lift it off and replace it without having to rewrap it.

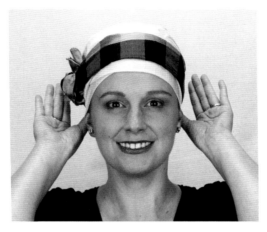

Tuck your thumbs up into it right behind your ears and slowly lift it off. I found that I could usually remove it and replace it at least three times before needing to unwrap it and start over again. The fact that you have no hair makes it very easy to do this.

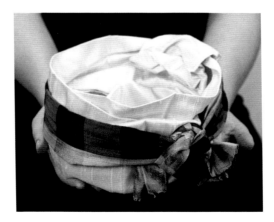

Great! Now we've covered the basic design for a simple Clochellay. But before I go on to the many different styles you can create, let's go over a quick list of "Don'ts."

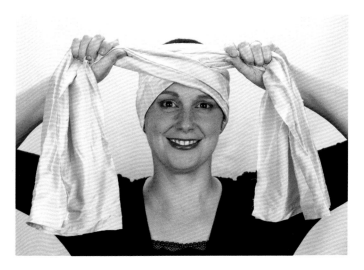

Don't #1: Make sure you don't cover your ears completely with the wrap and then leave it that way, or bunch it up so it's more like a wreath around your head. You need to allow the material to be wide enough so that it's crossing your forehead an inch or so above the eyebrows, covering the tips of the ears, and near enough to the crown of your head so you can tug the material over without too much effort.

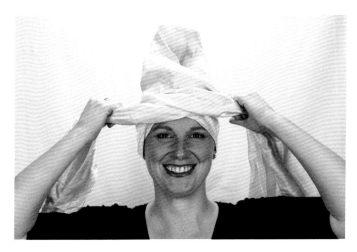

Don't #2: Don't allow the material in the back to point up at the top of your head! Not only will you look...um...*ridiculous*...but you'll not be able to tug the top material over to the other side without problems. The way it's wrapped in this photo shows three mistakes: too bunched, covering the ears completely, and not close enough to the crown on top.

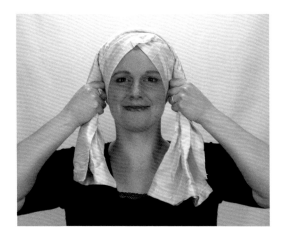

And, finally, *Don't #3*: Don't, under any circumstances, step out of the house with your Clochellay looking like this in the very front. This look *might* have worked for Gloria Swanson in the film *Sunset Boulevard*, but it's certainly not the look *we're* going for. Just remember: If you look like you're going out wearing a towel after you've just washed your hair, you've got it wrong! Back to the mirror with you!

Got it? Great! Now, take a look at the following link to see a how-to video of me wrapping this first basic style, just to be certain!

That's a Wrap Demonstration: http://vimeo.com/56447644.

Okay. Let's start playing with some of the many ways you can work with this basic wrap design on any particular day!

CHAPTER 4: VARIATIONS ON A THEME

The time that I expected to be bald was to be from early summer into the fall, so I knew I was going to need colors to go with those two seasons of my wardrobe. Remember to use the calculations for your swatch of material, which I explained in Chapter 1.

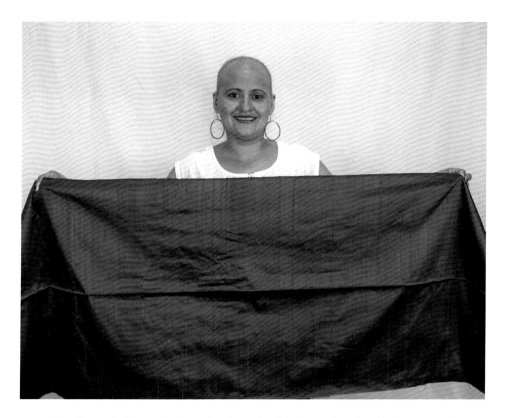

Here, Teresa is demonstrating what turned out to be my favorite shade—a swatch of chocolate brown Dupioni.

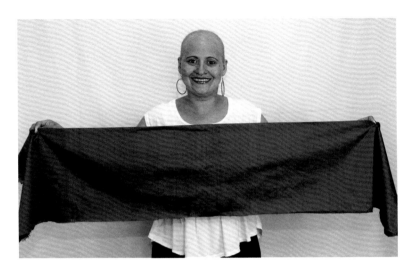

First, you fold it in half length-wise.

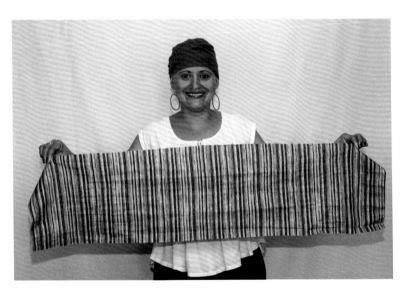

This time, I'm using a fun, striped accent wrap in browns, greens, and turquoise.

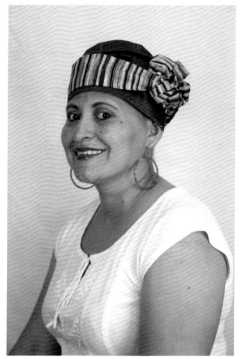 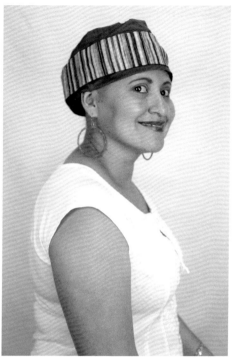

Here's how it looks when it's all put together, following the same steps as in Chapter 2.

I think that the darker base wraps, matched with a great accent material, are really appealing. But, who knows what you might come up with? Get creative with your colors and your wardrobe!

So, now you've got the basic technique. Let's try a couple more and then build on that.

DESIGN #3

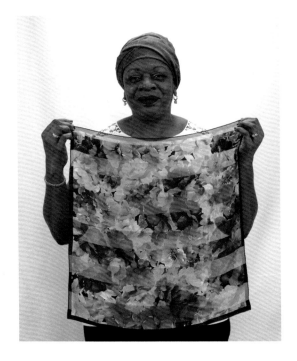

This silk scarf measures 21 inches square.

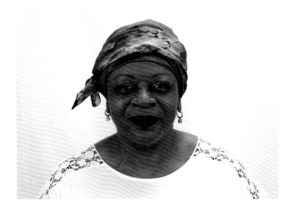

It's folded several times from the corners to make the width about 21½ inches. Then I just tied it on the side.

Go and peruse your scarf collection—you might be surprised at what you find that was too small to use alone, but which works wonderfully as an accent piece! Or, ask friends if you can borrow their scarves while you are going through this challenge. You'll be amazed at what starts coming your way.

DESIGN #4

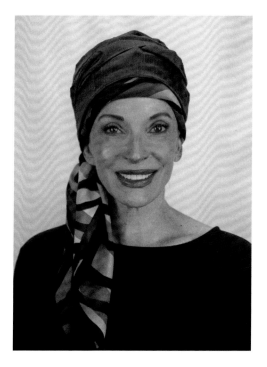

This fun animal print scarf measures 35 inches square. Again, I folded it from corner to corner until it was about 3 inches wide. I tied it once just behind my ear to let it hang for a "hair-like" feel and a more dramatic look.

But I could have tied it into a floppy bow, or even a half-bow. A bow on a scarf this large just gives it more volume on the side.

All right. At this point, you've learned the basic way to wrap a Clochellay, and several variations that you can do with it. Next, we'll be moving on to creating more styles that you can work with. But, before we do, I want to share this thought with you.

You might read some of these directions and think, "Wrap the what, *where*? Tie the which one, *when*?" Especially if you're going through chemo or radiation, you may find your brain to be a bit fuzzy these days.

So, please, don't worry if it takes you a couple of attempts (or four or five) to get some of these designs right. Just read the directions slowly and give yourself room for mistakes. Don't judge yourself if you have to do a bit of trial and error. I promise that you'll soon get the knack of it, and that people will be asking you, "How did you *do* that?"

That being said, let's move on!

DESIGN #5

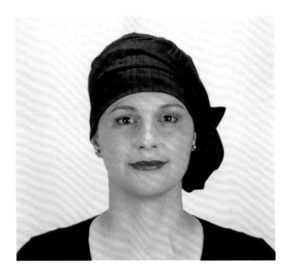

This time I used a black base and, rather than starting the base wrap exactly in the middle of the back of your head, I positioned the middle of the folded base-wrap material a couple of inches off to one side (it doesn't matter which side). This will enable you to tie the two ends behind one of your ears, leaving them untucked. The black base I used has iron-on hem tape at the ends and, once tied, I folded these ends over at the edges to give them a little more definition. Because the hem tape gives the ends more rigidity, it allows you to play with them, and they still stay put.

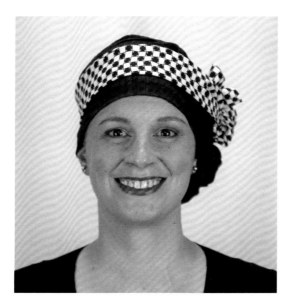

Then I wrapped a dynamic black-and-white patterned accent and arranged the ends above the same ear by pushing them into the accent band as we've done before.

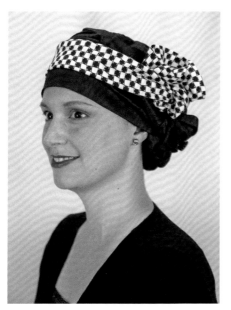
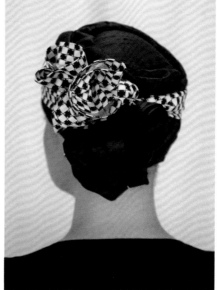

Here's the side view...and here's the back. This is one of my favorite styles!

Notice how I didn't tie off the base wrap and the accent wrap directly on top of each other? Being a little bit angled, as they are, gives a more elegant look.

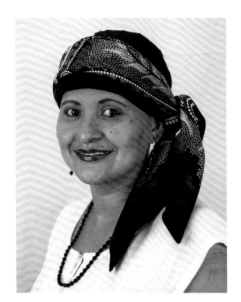 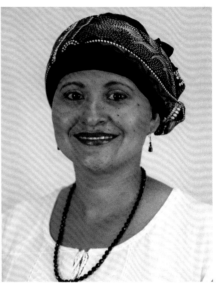

This next accent scarf measures 35 inches square—like the animal print that was previously demonstrated. You can leave it hanging...or you can tuck it in, as I've done with some of the other accent wraps.

You can see how I just wove it around and tucked and played with it to get a nice little bouffe on the side. By the way, if your accent scarf doesn't want to stay put when you do this, it's because you haven't tied it tightly enough around your head. If it's tight, it should stay put without any problems.

The way that you'll begin to have fun with any of these styles is to try different variations yourself. Let it hang loose one day, tie it up into a half-bow the next, and tuck it in completely the day after that.

Think about it—when you have hair, you probably only style it in a couple of different ways. But, scarves and wraps give you the advantage of being able to diversify! Now's your time to try myriad looks before your hair comes back in again and you have to stick with one short "do" for a while.

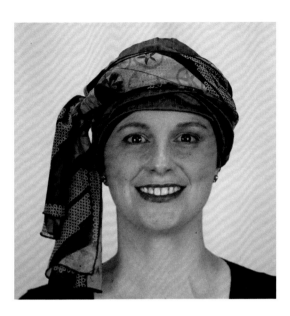

Here's another variation with a base wrap in a solid color. This blue is great because it goes well with black, as well as with light blue jeans. The accent scarf was so lightweight and long that I just tied it once and let it hang down.

Are you beginning to get the idea here? It makes a big difference in your look when you start with a Clochellay base and *then* add either an accent wrap or a scarf of your own! To see the difference, let's look in on what some women might consider their only option for a scarf measuring 41 inches square:

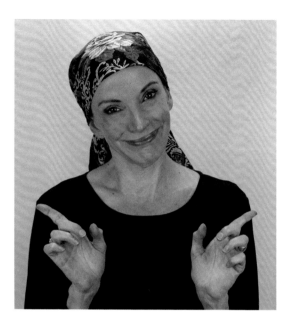

It isn't awful, but you *can* create something that's so much more flattering!

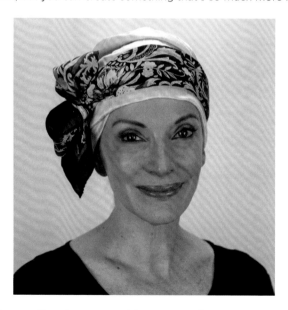

What a difference it makes to use this great scarf as an accent wrap instead, starting with a white Dupioni base.

I tied this with one of those "half-bows" I mentioned earlier, and I think it makes for a nice look. Not dome-headed, not too much frou-frou. Sure, people will still know that something's going on with your hair, but it's such a prettier look than the scarf alone.

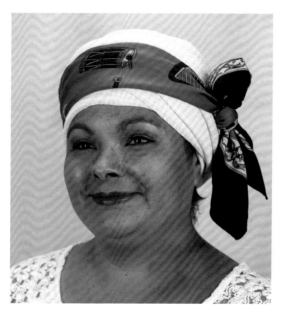

Here's how it looks with a yellow cotton base and a different accent scarf.

Beautiful, right? And, remember this: When you're out and about, surrounded by women with gorgeous hair, you have absolutely *no* idea who among them was bald at one point in their lives just as you are now. Survivors are everywhere! You just can't tell because their hair has grown back. That being said, let's talk about some more design options.

DESIGN #6

This time, we're going to mix it up a little and tie the accent wrap first. This blue scarf measures 11 inches x 53 inches.

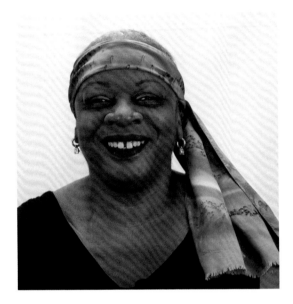

You start by folding the scarf in half so it's about 5½ inches in width, and then place the middle of the scarf at one side of your head, above your ear.

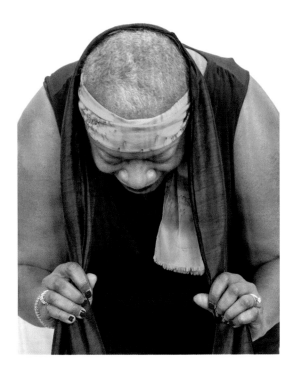

Allowing the blue ends to dangle down, take one of your base materials that goes well with your accent scarf, and wrap it like it was shown in the previous chapters, beginning in the back with the folded edge at the nape of your neck. Make sure that when you wrap the base wrap in the front, you allow the material of your scarf to peek out all across your forehead, adding color.

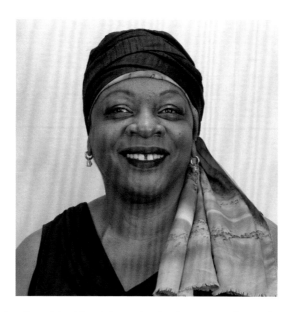

After wrapping it and tucking it in at the back, you can leave the ends of your scarf dangling like this, giving you that "long hair" feel...or you can do a couple of other things. One option is to tie it in the half-bow we talked about earlier.

DESIGN #7

Or, here's an idea: Take the two loose scarf ends and tuck them in at the top of your base wrap.

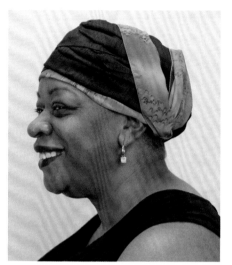 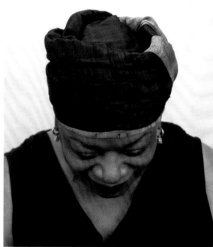

Here is a side and top view.

DESIGN #8

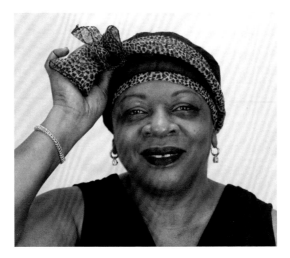

Take the two dangling ends and bring one around the front and the other around the upper portion of the back. This time I selected an animal print for the accent wrap.

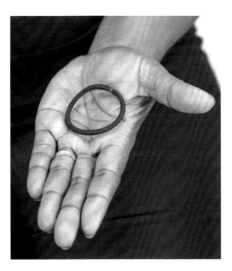

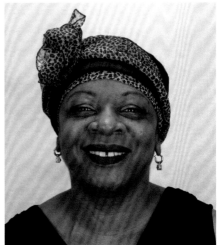

Then you can either take a plastic clip, or a covered band, like this one. Secure the two ends in place with the covered rubber band or with the clip on the other side of your head, as we did here.

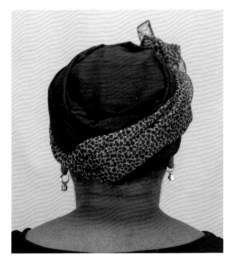 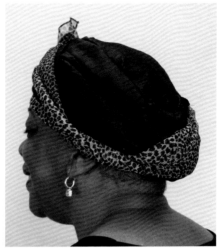

Here's how it looks in the back and from the side.

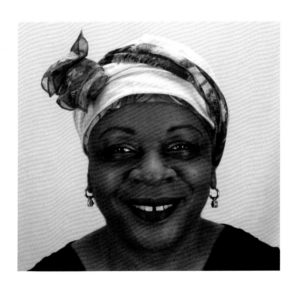

And here's what it would look like if you use lighter colors. Very pretty!

Remember that you can always tuck it into the top edge like before if you don't want to clip it and have that little frou-frou piece on the side.

DESIGN #9

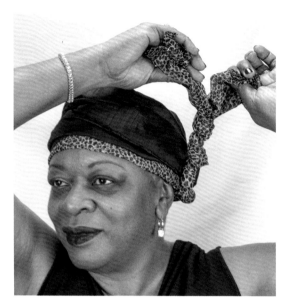

Twist the loose scarf ends together.

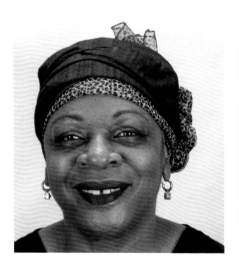
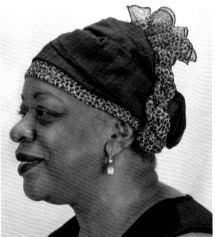

Then stick the ends down into the top fold of your base wrap—just enough to hold it in place, yet still allowing the very ends of the scarf to stick out, giving it a little flair. I really like this one.

DESIGN #10

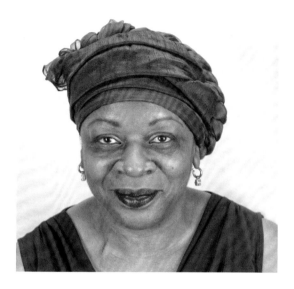

You can create another version by using a longer accent scarf and pulling it all the way across the top of your head to the other side before tucking it into the side of the base wrap. This orange scarf measures 10 inches x 60 inches.

You can also create this using the accent wrap on the outside of the base wrap. Just wrap it once around the base wrap, as always, and then tie the ends behind the back of one of your ears. Next, twist the ends together and proceed as in **Design #9**.

DESIGN #11

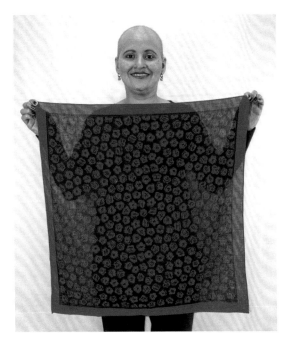

This scarf measures 26 inches square. Fold it into a triangle and place it with the folded side down at the middle of the back of your head, allowing the front corner of the material to dangle over one eye.

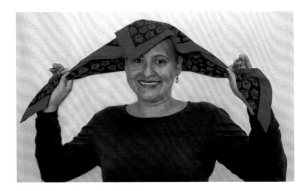

Then take the corners (as the model is holding in her hands) and tie them together at your forehead, above the other eye. You want to make sure and tie it so that the points of the scarf that are hanging over your eye are now underneath the tied part. See?

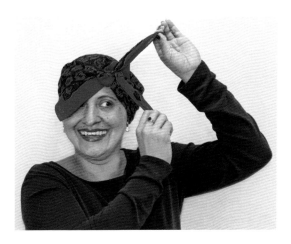

Now, wrap your base wraps over it, allowing the parts I just mentioned to peek out from underneath at your forehead.

With this style, you don't have to "tug" the top part over to cover your crown because it's already covered with the first scarf that you tied.

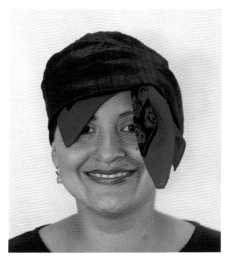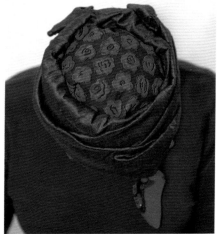

Now, take the two end dangling parts that are hanging down over one of your eyes, lift them up, and tuck them into the base wrap.

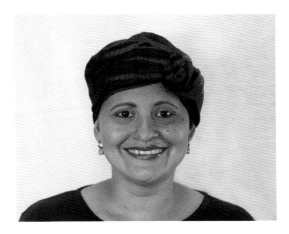

After that, you'll take the other pointed end of the scarf that you left dangling over one of your eyes and tuck it up under the base wrap just enough for the edge of it to still show, as shown in the photo.

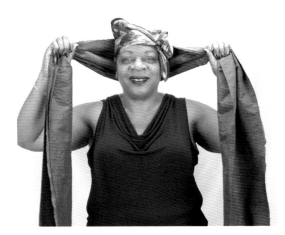

This piece of Dupioni measures 96 inches x 22 inches. I'm going for a more dramatic look this time.

I created another variation on this design by using a smaller accent wrap and a longer base wrap. The accent wrap in this photo measures 24 inches square. I tied it as I did in **Design #11**, only, this time, when it's folded from corner to corner into a triangle and then tied from the back of the head, only the ends will be long enough to hang down in your face. Tie those ends at one of your temples.

Let's start it in the back with the folded edge at the nape of your neck—just like a normal base wrap—but, because it's so long, we'll end up tying it at completion in the front.

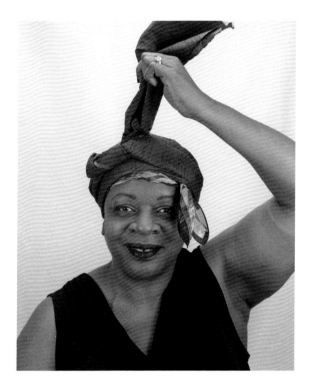

Wrap it around your forehead (allowing the two tie ends of the accent scarf to dangle down) and then around to the back and secure it with a half-knot. Then bring it back around to above the temple in the front and tie it once. At this point, you'll tuck the ends into its own folds. I also made sure to allow the front floral scarf to show all across the model's forehead. This photo shows how it's tucked into the base wrap above the temple.

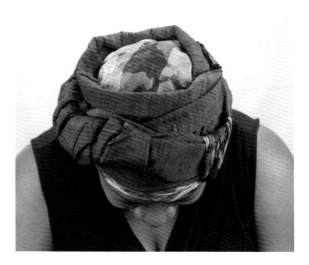

Again, the top is taken care of by the first, smaller scarf.

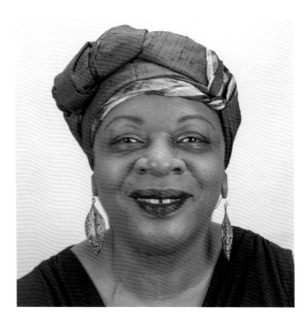

Next, pull up the little tie parts of the accent wrap that are dangling and tuck them into the base wrap. This is a great style when you want just a hint of an accent color, but of course, you can try this style with the longer base wrap alone. That's beautiful too!

DESIGN #12

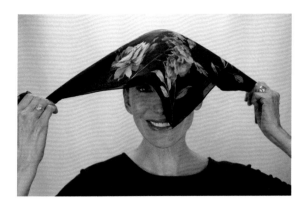

Here, I'm using a smaller scarf than the previous two, measuring 21 inches square. Fold it at opposite corners to make a triangle—this time leaving the two loose corner points hanging down *over one of your nostrils,* as opposed to hanging over an eye, and tie it in the back.

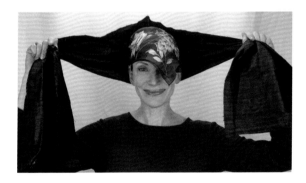

Then take one of your base wraps and wrap it just as we did earlier, with the fold at the nape of your neck. Make sure to cover the two tie-ends of the accent wrap at the back of your head.

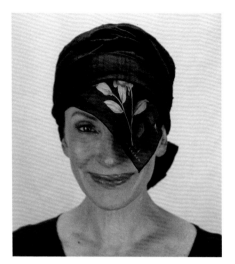 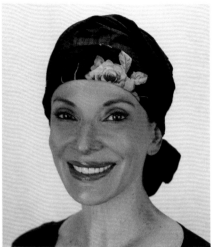

Once you get the base wrap in place, gently tug the two tie-ends of the base wrap over toward the same side of your head as your dangling scarf (so they are near the back of your ear) and tie them once. Don't tuck them in this time so they'll show just a little bit from the front-view, as seen in the photo. Next, you'll pull up the dangling corners of the accent wrap and tuck them into the base wrap.

I like the way this one looks because I used a black base with a black background accent wrap, and they blend so it looks like it's just one piece of material.

DESIGN #13

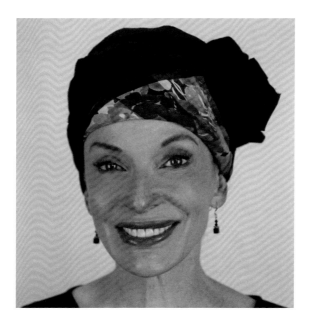

This wrap is a lot like the previous design, except the base wrap is finished much higher on the side. In order to do this, begin by wrapping the accent scarf as you did in **Design #11**, allowing the front corners to drape over one eye. As you begin tying the base wrap, instead of placing the center of the base wrap at the back of your head, start with its center at the *side* of your head, just behind one of your ears (the same side as the accent scarf dangling over one eye). When it's finished, the two end pieces will land just behind and above one of your ears.

In this design, you'll tie the ends once, and then you'll take a covered band and wrap it two or three times around the end pieces. Once secured, you should be able to tweak the edges, folding them under if you like to make a pretty bouffe. You may have to push the base wrap around a bit so you can place the bouffe just above and behind the ear, but no worries. The base wrap is very forgiving if you need to adjust it a bit!

Then you pull up the portion of the scarf that's draped over one eye and tuck it into the base wrap. That's all there is to it!

DESIGN #14

Up until this point, I've been using various scarves underneath the base wraps. This time, I'm going to show you what you can do using one of the accent pieces you purchased.

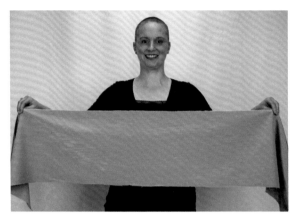

For **Design #14**, you'll put the accent piece on first as an under-color.

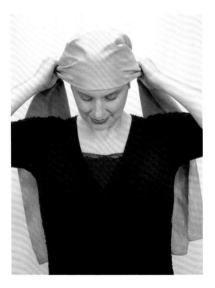

The only portion of the accent wrap you'll fold this time is the edge that you'll place at your forehead—just to ensure that it's smooth and has no strings dangling. Begin by wrapping it from the front to the back.

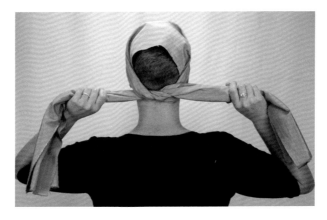

Tie it once in the back and bring the remainder of it to the front again.

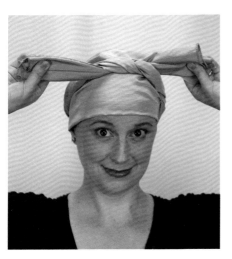 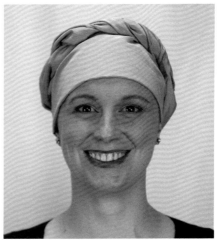

Tie it once in the front, up near the crown of your head, and then tuck in the loose ends. (The model wound the ends around the blue material once more and then tucked them in to give it a "woven look," as seen in the photo.) You want the part that's tied in front to be a bit high because the base wrap is going to fit beneath it.

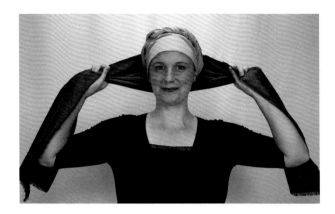

Start the base wrap in the back, with the folded edge at the nape of your neck, as you normally do. Wrap it as before, with the fabric wrapped smoothly across your forehead and an inch or two above your eyebrows. This time, however, make sure that the tied portion of the accent wrap can be seen above your base wrap.

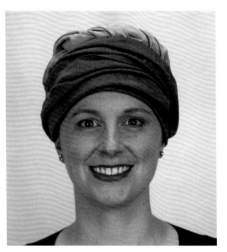 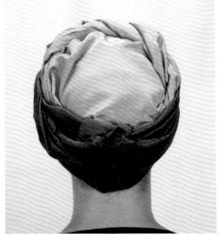

After it's wrapped around the front and tucked in at the back, it will look something like it does in the photo. You don't have to worry about tugging the top over on this one because the accent wrap is already covering your crown. See how the blue wrap near the crown gives your head a little volume? This is another favorite of mine.

DESIGN #15

Even though I highly recommend Dupioni for your main base wraps (and I think you'll find that Dupioni will end up being your favorite fabric), you can use other fabrics as long as they are malleable, comfortable, and not too slippery on your skin.

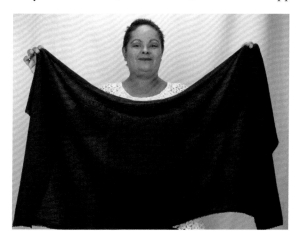

This time, we're going to use a piece of black muslin measuring 56 inches x 22 inches. Fold it in half and wrap it just like a regular base wrap. Muslin doesn't hold its shape as well as Dupioni, but it still does a pretty good job, and it's very soft!

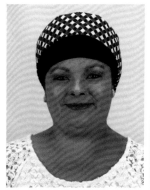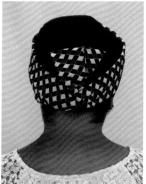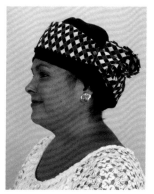

As before, tug the black muslin over to cover the top of your head. Then you'll take an accent wrap and fold it lengthwise into thirds. Wrap it as shown in the photo, starting with the middle of the accent wrap high up on the forehead and bringing it around to the back, tying it once, and then tucking it into itself.

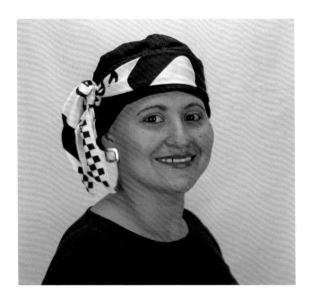

By the way, elongated scarves that measure 7 inches x 32 inches, like this black-and-white scarf, make particularly wonderful accent wraps. This is a size I like to tie twice at the side, and then let the remaining material hang loose.

DESIGN #16

This is going to sound like something we've already done, but stay with me, as it *is* different. This time, I'll start with a white Dupioni base wrap with hemmed edges at the ends.

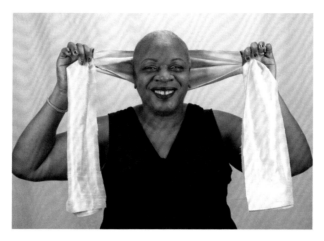

Begin by wrapping the Clochellay as you'd normally wrap a base wrap, except that you'll start by placing the middle of the base material at a point just behind one of your ears.

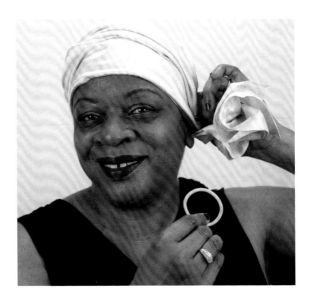

You're doing this because you want the ends to land right behind your earlobe, near the base of your skull, where you'll secure the ends with a covered band.

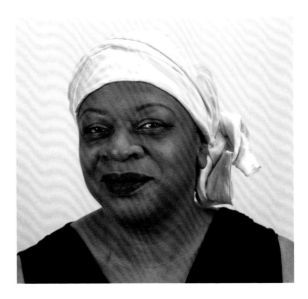

Don't forget to tug the top part over the crown of your head.

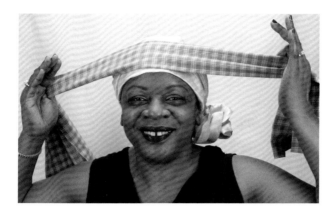

Next, take one of your accent wraps, folded into thirds or fourths length-wise, and start wrapping it with the middle a little off to the side in front (the opposite side from the bouffe) so that its ends will meet up with your base wrap ends— behind your ear.

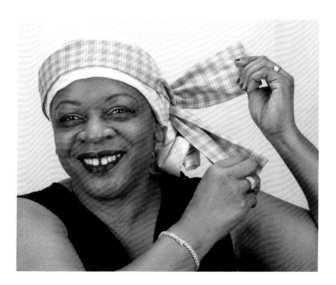

Tie the ends twice, or three times if you have a bit too much material. Then fluff the loose ends until you get them as you want them. You might want to fold the edges over to give them more volume, but make sure they are hemmed with hem-tape or they won't have any body to them.

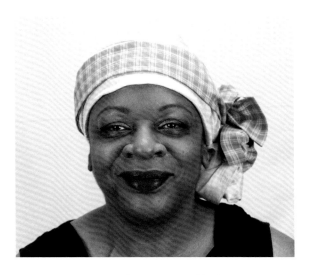

This one is fun and casual looking!

DESIGN #17

This time, we'll create a wrap the same as with the white silk base wrap that was in the previous design, only we'll start with one of the accent wraps to give it a little color underneath.

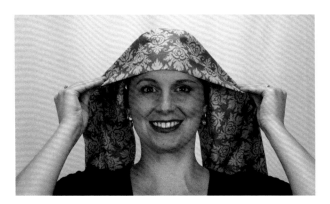

Don't fold it in thirds lengthwise; just fold the part that covers your forehead over a bit so it's not frayed. Then tie it in the back and tuck the ends into the folds of the material.

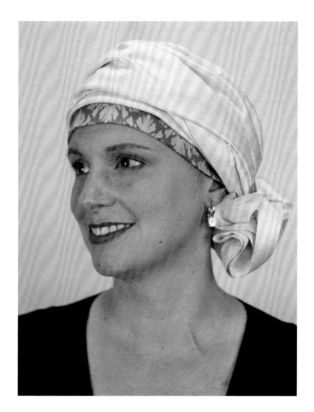

Next, wrap your base wrap over it, beginning with the middle of the base wrap just behind one ear as in the previous design (but going a little higher on your forehead than you normally would to allow the blue accent wrap to show), tug the top across to cover your crown, and then tie the ends together with the ponytail band so the ends land behind your earlobe. Then fluff the ends by folding the hemmed edges. Nice, right?

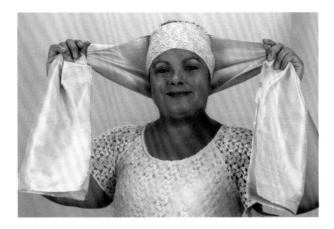

Let's do another version of this style. It's wrapped the same as we've been doing in the two previous designs, only, this time, you want to end up with the bouffe *above* your ear. Start by wrapping an accent piece flat across your forehead with the edge tucked under, tying and tucking it in back. Then begin wrapping your base wrap on top of the accent piece, positioning the middle of the base material directly at the side of your head as in **Designs #15** and **#16**. But this time, you want to end up with the ends *above* the ear when you finish.

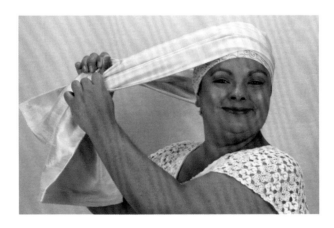

Make sure you let the accent wrap show at your forehead. Don't cover it up! Now take those two loose ends that are located directly above your ear and secure them with a covered ponytail band.

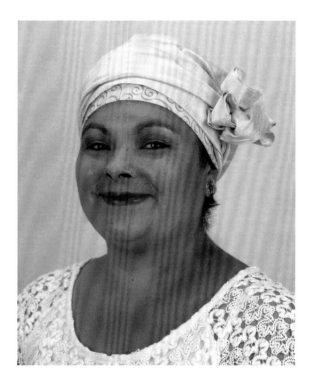

Once you have them held in place, work with the ends until you mold them into the shape you want. Remember, you must have hem tape to accomplish this!

DESIGN #18

This is a very elegant style that can pop with lots of color.

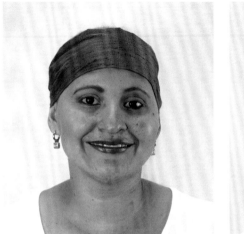 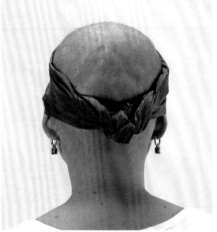

With this design, start with an accent material at your forehead, as we've done previously. Then wrap a base wrap the regular way and tuck it into itself at the back.

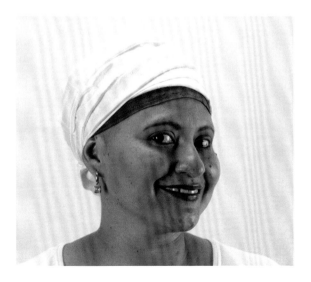

Wrap your base wrap over that.

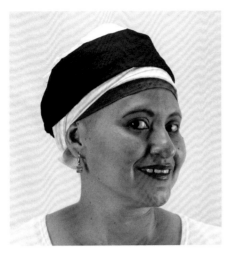 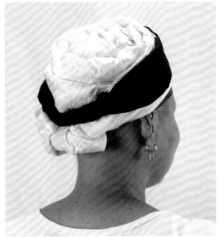

After that, add one more accent wrap over the base wrap just for extra color. See how wonderful the Dupioni looks as an accent wrap?

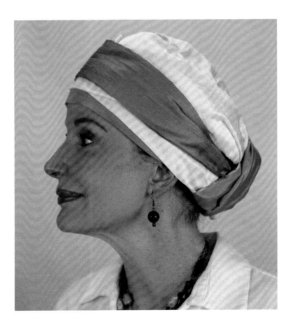

Here it is in different accent colors, except for one little change—I didn't tuck it into the first base wrap. Instead, I pulled the two tie ends up and tucked them higher in the back for this one.

DESIGN #19

Now, we're going to move on to something really different. I started with a gauzy scarf measuring 18 inches x 63 inches, though it doesn't have to be gauzy. Just make sure it's very long and lightweight for this particular design.

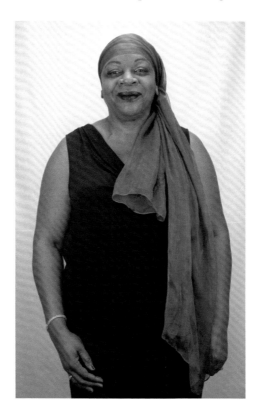

Fold the material in half length-wise (with the folded edge at your forehead) and wrap it from the front to the back of your head, tying it behind one of your ears so one end is about 8 inches longer than the other end.

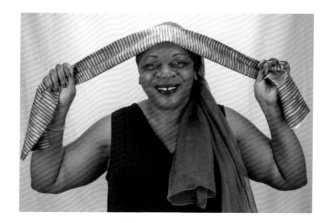

Then take one of your accent wraps, fold it into thirds or fourths as usual, and, beginning rather high and in the front, bring it around to the back of your head and tie it, tucking the ends into itself afterward.

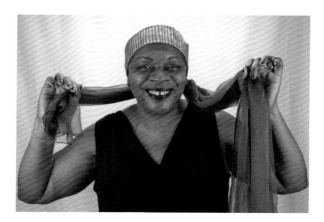

Take the two ends in your hands and twist the material a bit so it doesn't hang too loosely. Then take the shorter piece and bring it around from the back of your head and over your forehead toward your opposite ear so it's now wrapped around three-quarters of your head.

Take the longer piece from the back and wrap it around to the front of your head, as well (heading in the opposite direction of your first, shorter piece), but then, continue around the back and toward the side again so the two ends can meet. This longer piece will have wrapped around your head one-and-a-quarter times. And, wherever the two ends meet is fine, as long as it's somewhere off to the side. Play with it until it hits the right spot for you.

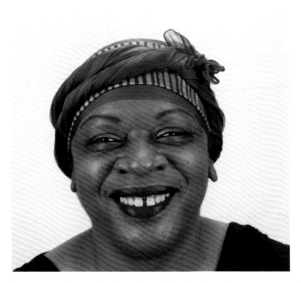

Once the two ends are both at the side, tie them into a square knot.

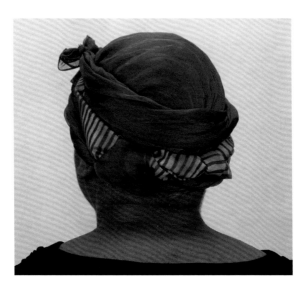

Here's how it looks from the back. People often stopped and asked me about this one. They seemed to really like it, and so did I! It's unusual.

DESIGN #20

For another option, instead of wrapping the two long ends around your head until the ends meet with just enough to tie them together, you'll wrap the longest end around the back of your head, past your ear, and then over the front of your head, so it encircles your head only once, as in this photo.

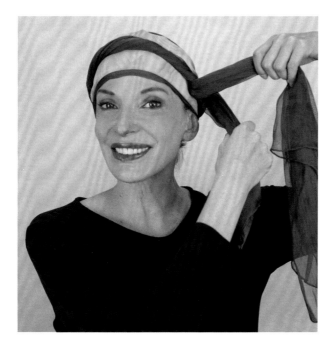

Tie the ends once at the side of your head and then begin twisting them.

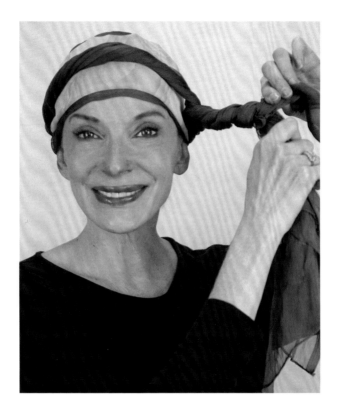

Soon, they'll be twisted to the point they'll begin bending.

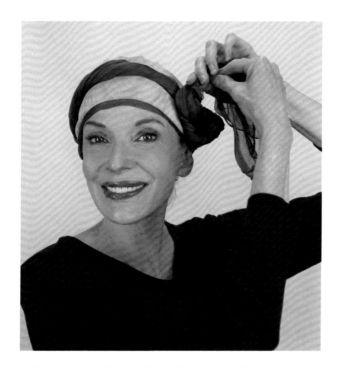

Keep twisting and use the bending of the material to wrap them into a small flower at the side of your head. You'll want to tie the ends together to keep the twist in place once you tuck it in.

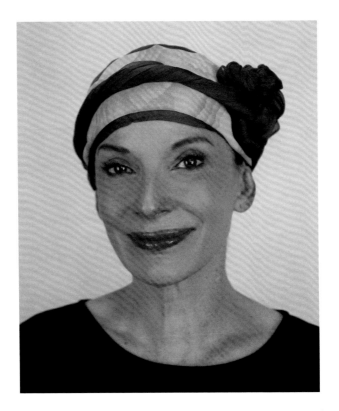

Then tuck in the ends and, *voila*—you have another great look!

Now let's move on to a completely new design.

CHAPTER 5: THERE'S MORE THAN ONE WAY TO WRAP A HEAD

During the months while I was having fun experimenting with various ways to cover my tressless head, I dreamed up the following version one night while lying awake around 2:30 a.m. I got up and tried it the next day and, happily, it worked! I used white cotton seersucker, which is also a nice material to use. (But, Dupioni is still, in my opinion, the best.)

DESIGN #21

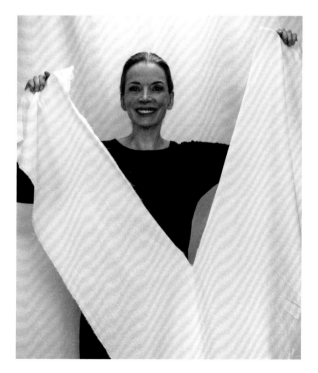

Take a piece of base material that has the initial beginning measurements we discussed in Chapter 1. Mine was 44 inches x 58 inches before I cut it lengthwise. Cut the material towards the middle of the fabric length-wise, but *stop*, leaving about six inches un-cut in the very center of the midline.

This time, we're not going to cut the original piece of material in two, creating two separate base wraps. This time, you'll only have one wrap from your original piece of material.

FYI, this base wrap is going to have twice the bulk around your head as the ones we've done previously, since we're using *all* of the material instead of cutting it in half. This is nice, since there are times when you may want a fuller look.

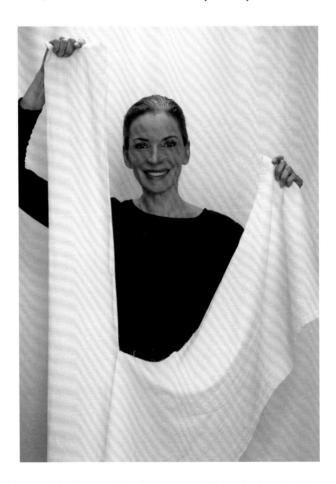

Next, fold *one* of the large strips of the material length-wise. Don't worry about the other strip, as we'll get to that later. This design takes a little practice, by the way, but once you understand how it works, it's really easy to do!

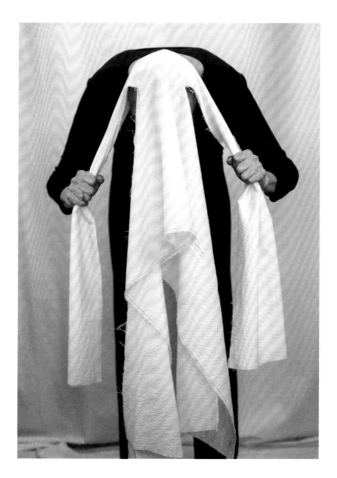

You'll begin to wrap it around your head just like before, with the one folded edge toward the nape of your neck.

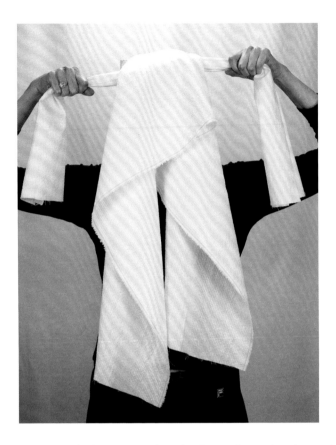

Wrap the back folded pieces around to the front of your head, crossing over each other at the forehead as we've done before, and then straighten up, as shown in the photo.

Note that the two pieces I have in my hands are about to be tied in the back, *not* brought around to the front again. They are already crossed across my forehead at the front, underneath the hanging piece of material. So, now, I'll tie them in the back.

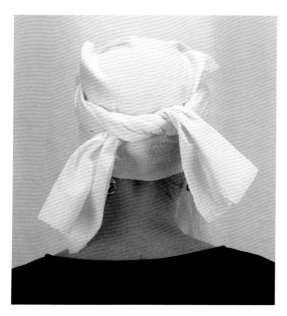

Here's what the knot looks like when it's been tied once in the back. Just leave the two end pieces untucked for now. Next, we'll deal with the front.

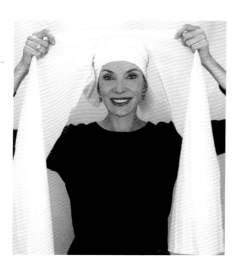 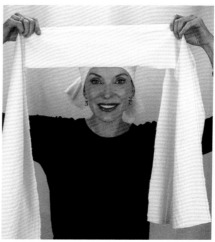

You can see when I lift up the front piece that I crossed the first piece of the base wrap over my forehead, just like a normal base wrap. Now, take this loose-hanging front piece and fold it back onto itself lengthwise like we originally folded the first piece.

Once you've folded it, pull it flat so you don't have a puff of material at the top of your head. The wider you fold the second piece of base wrap, the flatter the top part will be. Just try this a couple of times and you'll understand what I'm talking about.

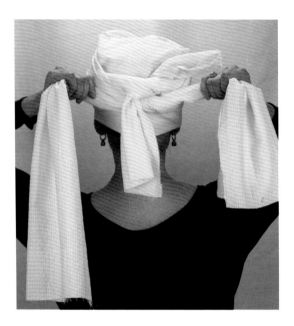

Once it's folded and pulled flat, bring the ends around to the back, but don't stop and tie them there! Wrap them around again toward the front, where you will *now* tie them once.

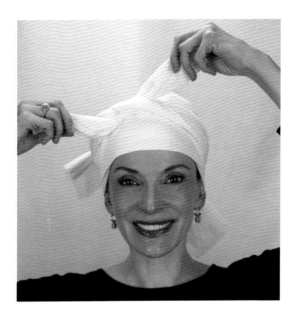

Make sure you tie the ends kind of high in front to give you a nice lift. This way, you also have room to place an accent piece right by your face.

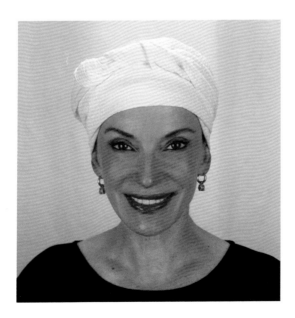

This is the point at which you tuck in all the ends—both front and back.

Remember: There's no need to tug over the top on this one! It's already covered.

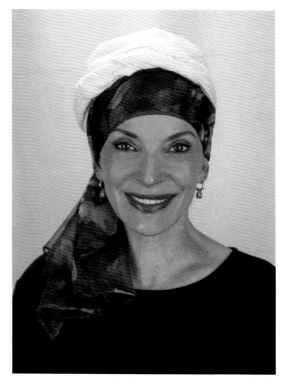

Now, take one of your favorite accent wraps or scarves and fold it into thirds or fourths like we did in previous chapters. Wrap it near your face from the front to the back, tie it to the side, and leave the ends out—or tuck them in, if you like.

Well! We've covered a lot of varieties of what you can do for daytime Clochellays, so now we'll move on to some suggestions for an evening look. Just because you're temporarily tressless doesn't mean you can't look chic for an elegant event!

CHAPTER 6: EASY AND ELEGANT WRAPS FOR A DRESSY OCCASION

One of my concerns when I was without hair was what I would do in the case of attending a dressy affair. Would a Clochellay look good with a long, slinky dress? No, I felt that it was just a bit too daytime looking to wear with strappy stilettos. But not to fret, because here's something really elegant that you can do!

DESIGN #22

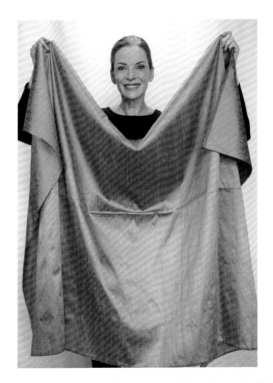

I highly recommend Dupioni for this one, as it has just the right amount of texture. The gold piece pictured measures 44 inches x 58 inches, the same as the others I purchased for base wraps, except, this time, I didn't cut it length-wise down the middle. I didn't use hem tape, either, as there is no need on this one. Everything will be tucked in.

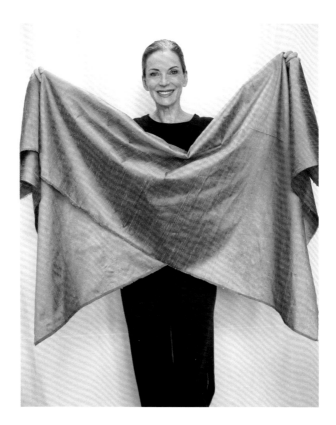

First, take the top left-hand corner and bottom right-hand corner of the material in your hands. This will cause it to fold over as shown in the photo. And, just a note—one of the main things you'll need here, besides the silk, is a little *courage*. It's going to seem cumbersome folding this one, and you'll feel like "I'm not doing it right!" But, have no fear and keep going. You'll be surprised how it all comes together in the end!

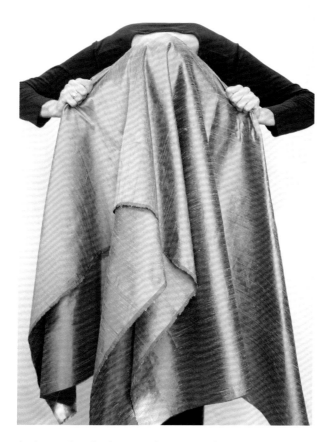

Lean over, inch your hands closer to the center of the material, and pull it tight.

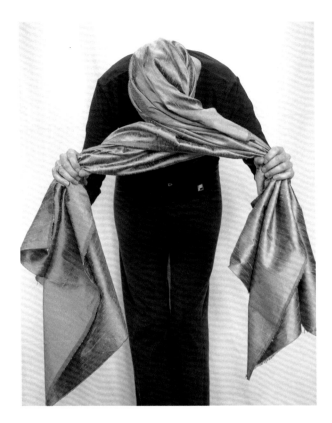

Cross the ends in front of your forehead as you always do. You'll probably have to really bunch the material up into each of your hands in order to cross it over in front.

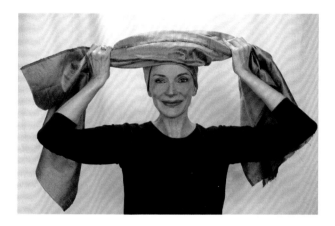

Then pull each of the crossed-over ends out to opposite sides of your head, straighten back up, and get yourself in front of a mirror!

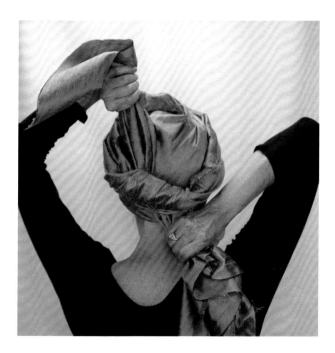

Bring both ends around to the back and cross them over once in a single knot.

Here's a perk! You don't have to worry about covering the top of your head this time because there's so much material, it'll automatically be covered.

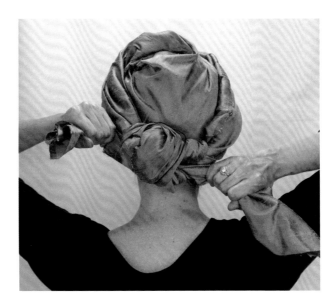

Now, tie the two ends once more so you've got a square knot. It doesn't really matter if it's a square one or not, as it's going to look great any way you tie it.

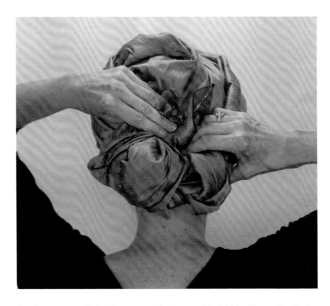

And, as a final step, tuck in those end pieces. But this time, tuck them both in somewhere upward in the wrap, instead of going underneath the material at the nape of the neck. With this much material, it's easy to find a place to stick those ends!

After you've got everything tucked in, you can begin to play with the material in the back—push it around, tucking in the edges until you get it into a shape you like. One of the best things about this particular style is it's very forgiving and quite malleable.

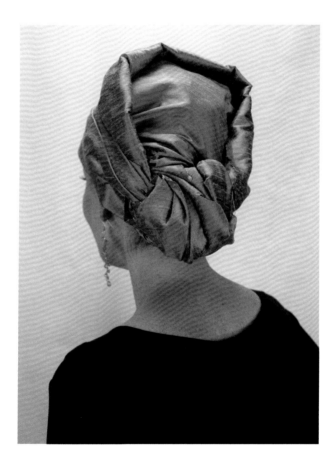

Here is how the back should look—or close to it—when you're finished. It looks almost like you're wearing a chignon of sorts, only made of material.

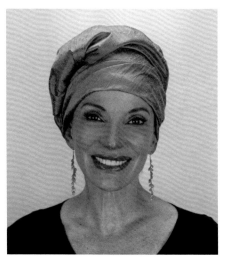 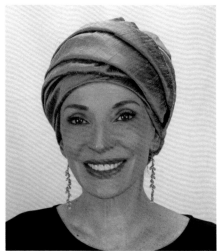

And, here is what the front will look like, give or take a few folds! I did this wrap twice and took photos to show that it can fall a different way each time you wrap it, and *every* way is correct!

Remember that you can push the top around as well until it's as low and subdued as you might like. Please don't be discouraged if you have to wrap it a couple of times before you like the way it looks. I have a feeling you'll surprise yourself, however, at how much you like it on the first try.

One of the nicest aspects of wearing this for an evening out is that, no matter the wind or weather (i.e., rain, drizzle, and so on), you'll still remain put-together looking. No worries about the possibilities of having a bad hair day when it comes to enjoying an elegant evening out!

DESIGN #23

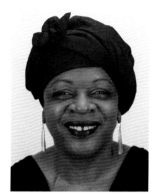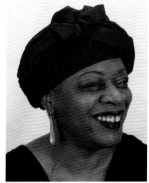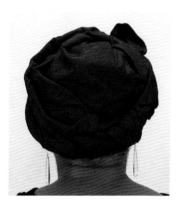

Here is another option in a gorgeous purple Dupioni that measures 44 inches x 75 inches. Instead of making the chignon in the back by tucking the ends in, the model brought them around to the front and tied them off to the side above an eye.

As I've mentioned earlier in the book, you can search for "gele wraps" online to see some amazing demonstrations. YouTubers can get pretty creative with those geles! You'll see that mine is a much more toned-down version, but watching a video or two online will help you understand what you can do with the right piece of textured material.

Now, let's move on to an easy, comfortable look for going to a ballgame or out and about running errands.

CHAPTER 7: CASUAL AND QUICK

Have you got a baseball cap? If so, you probably haven't felt much like wearing it since you lost your hair. Baseball caps aren't the best at covering all the surface we might like to bundle up when we're bald, especially around the back of the head.

However, there's a way to get around that problem and put that ball cap to use. All you need is a ball cap and a really long scarf.

DESIGN #24

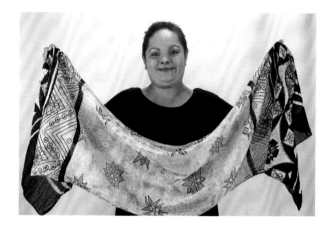

This cotton scarf measures 20 inches x 71 inches.

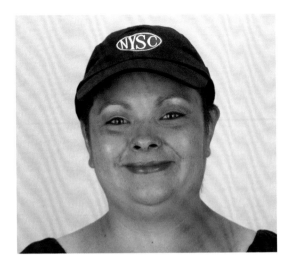

Now, take a look in your closet shelves and see if you can find a low-fitting baseball cap. **Important Note:** Caps that stick up high in the front will not work well for this design. So try to find a cap that fits low on the head, like the one in the photo.

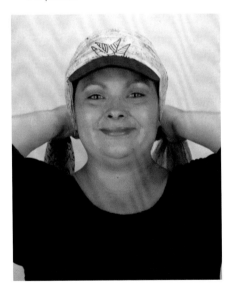
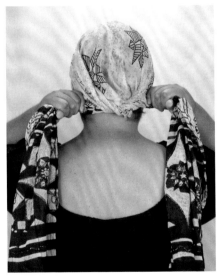

First, you don't fold the material. Just begin with the middle of the scarf at the front of the cap and wrap it around to the back, where you will tie it once.

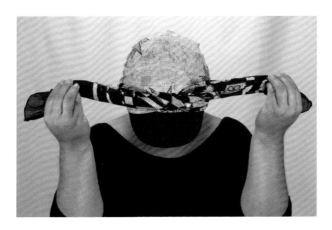

Then bring it back around to the front, where you will tie it once again at your crown. Now, bring it back around to the back a final time and tie it and tuck it in. If you don't have enough material to tie it, just tuck it in. Or, if you are using material that's a lot shorter than what I'm using here, just have the tie at the front be the final tie and tuck it in after that.

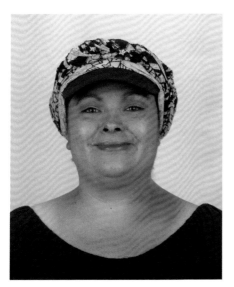
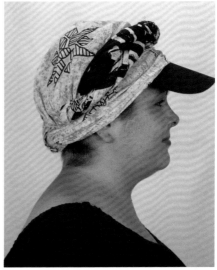

Now, you've got a more put-together look that covers a lot more than just a ball cap!

You can tug the back and sides down a bit for more coverage too. And, remember that this look is *great* for a bad hair day once those locks start to grow back in. But, if you're like me, there will be no more bad hair days for you—only *thankful-for-hair* days.

DESIGN # 25

Here's another super casual wrap that's really comfortable and only takes moments to do. This time, I'm using T-shirt material. It's so light and wraps very easily, yet it has nice texture to it so you still have some substance at the crown.

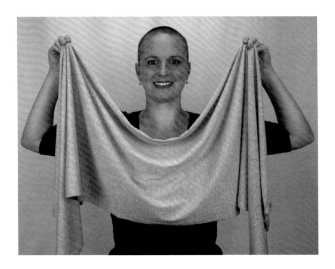

This gray swatch measures 68 inches x 18 inches.

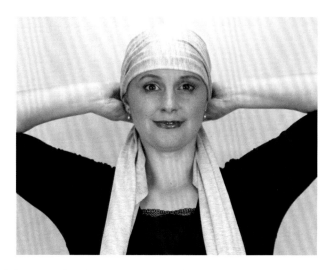

Just fold the part of it that's right at your forehead so you have a smooth edge with no fraying showing. One-third of the "end tail" should be in your right hand and two-thirds of the "end tail" should be in your left hand.

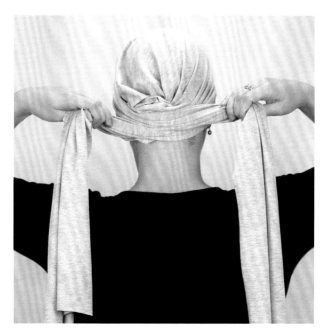

Cross them over in the back. Do not tie them!

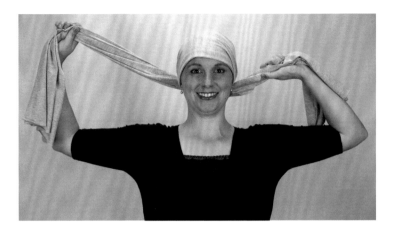

Now, you'll want to maneuver the material (it will slide on your skin) so the tails have a ratio of one-third in your left hand to two-thirds in your right. After you wrap it across in the back, you'll bring the long part in your right hand across your forehead and over to the other tail that you're holding in your left hand so they meet right behind your left ear and are approximately the same length. If the ratio isn't quite right when you land behind your left ear, you can still slide the material around until they are about even.

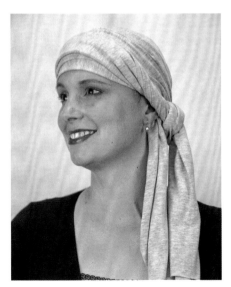

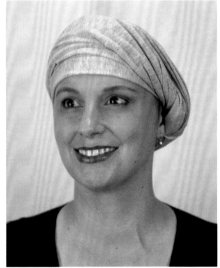

Once it's at the side of your head, tie it in a half-knot. You can wear it dangling... or you can tuck in the ends in the back. It looks great that way too.

DESIGN #26

If you want, you can add an accent wrap.

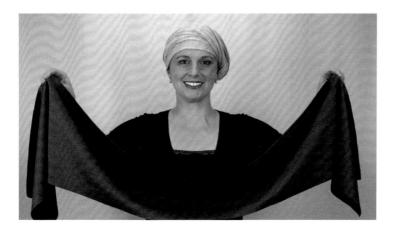

This dark gray swatch is also T-shirt material that measures 9 inches x 68 inches.

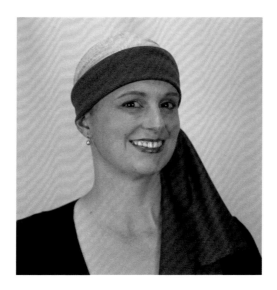

I folded the darker gray material in thirds length-wise, started wrapping it with the center of the material over one eyes (so the ends will be even when it's tied behind one ear), and then tied it in a square knot. This looks really great to be so quick and comfortable, doesn't it?

DESIGN #27

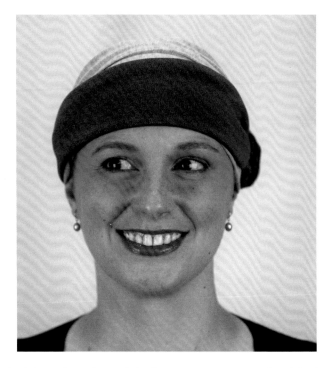

You can let it hang for a dramatic look, or you can wrap and tuck in the ends as shown here in **Design #27**.

Important Tip: Depending on the circumference of your head, you might want to trim the ends so they are a little bit shorter if you want to wrap and tuck them.

DESIGN #28

I've created two final, easy, quick, and super casual head wraps for **Designs #28** and **#29**. These don't fall under the category of Clochellay, since Clochellays are created by wrapping open-ended material. But, they're such easy-to-do, great-looking, and inexpensive wraps that I just had to include them.

They use T-shirt material as well, only *this* time you actually *harvest* the material from a T-shirt!

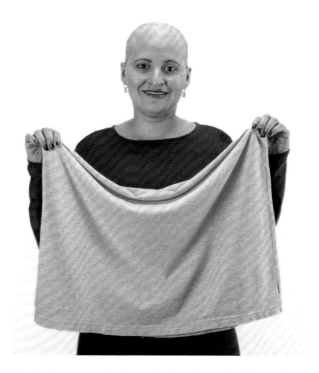

Take a T-shirt, sized large or extra-large, that you're ready to toss. (Goodwill is great for finding all sorts of sizes and colors at low prices). Cut it straight across the chest, starting at just below the armpit seam. I used an old gray T-shirt, size large.

Important Tip: If you have a small head, a medium-sized T-shirt might even work.

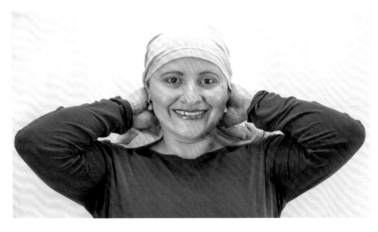

Place the "circle" of material around your head with a portion of the hemmed edge at your forehead.

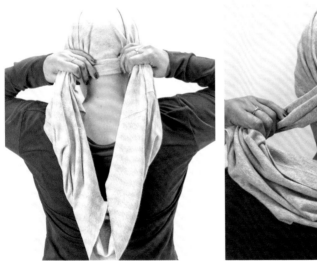
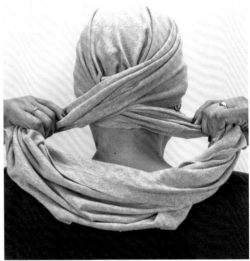

Pull the rest of the material behind your head...and cross it over once, at the nape of your neck. This will create a loop that you're holding in your hands. Next, you're going to place this loop back onto your head, like a bandeau.

Important Tip: If the loop is too large to fit snugly on your head, you may need to cross the end pieces of material over once more, as the model did.

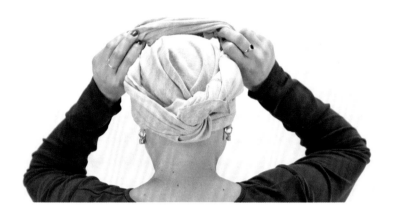

Now, take the loop and pull it over your crown, securing the front of it high on your forehead. I'm going to call this loop the "Heidi Loop," because, once it's in place, it should resemble the braids that the storybook character, Heidi, used to wear crossed over the top of her head. Bring the Heidi Loop back over your head and pull it into place towards your forehead. You'll need to work with it a little bit to get it where you want it on your head while holding the portion of the T-shirt steady that's already covering your crown.

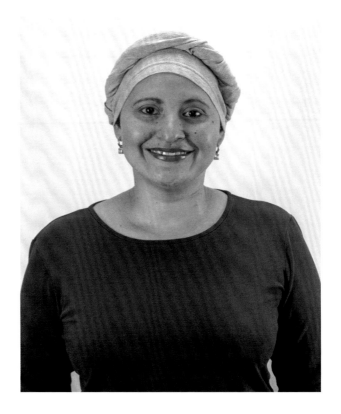

Now, tuck all the dangling bits under, working with the Heidi Loop until it has a fairly consistent thickness to it, much like wrapped braids would appear.

Voila! You're ready for the day! But, I say, *why stop there when adding one more thing can make it look even better?*

DESIGN #29

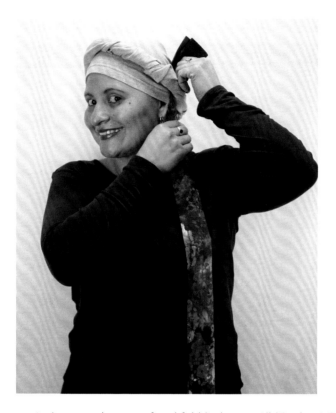

Take an accent piece or a long scarf and fold it down until it's about 2 inches wide. Tuck one end of the accent wrap into the Heidi Loop above your ear.

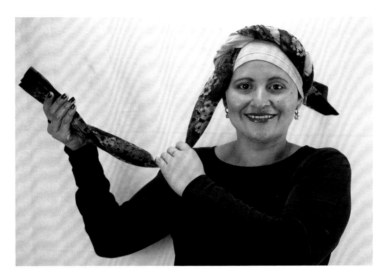

Next, take the accent piece and wind it around the Heidi Loop—circling your head—until you arrive back at the ear where you began.

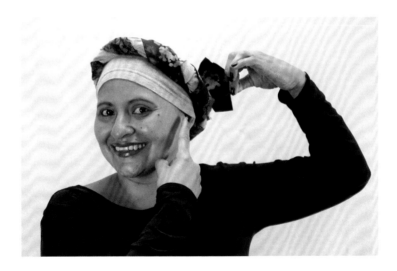

If you used an accent wrap that's at least 44 inches in length, there should be a few inches left over to create a little side bouffe, just to give it some flair!

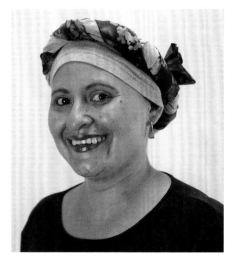 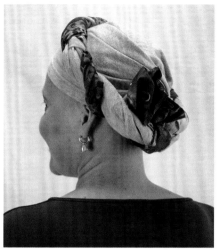

So, here's how it looks from the side and the back.

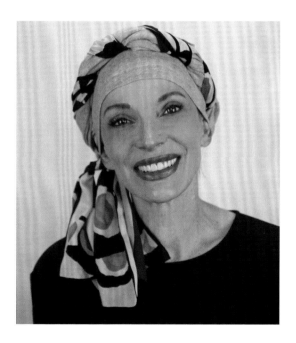

Here's how it looks with a long scarf woven through it.

You're going to receive compliments on this one, I promise. And, you'll also enjoy showing others how easy it is to create!

So, there you have it! Twenty-nine ways to wrap your head that will keep you looking your best as you're going through your time of being without hair.

It's my wish that you'll not only find these designs helpful, but that you'll also have as much fun working with them as I did. Wrapping fabric on your bald head, or in your hair once it's grown back, is a great style accessory. I know you'll look wonderful!

Now, go do something pretty with that beautiful head of yours. It's been great wrapping with you!

SOME FINAL THOUGHTS

So far, everything we've been talking about addresses the *external* matters regarding chemo-related hair loss. But, now that we've covered the 29-plus wrapping styles together, I'd like to take this opportunity to peer through the opposite end of the viewfinder—placing our focus on an *internal* consideration or two.

Look, I'm going to confess something. During the years I worked as an actress in Hollywood, I got a little caught up in the shallow end of the vanity pool. I had some collagen injected here and there. And, more than once, I laid down my hard-earned cash for the temporary tautness of some Botox. I colored my hair; I whitened my teeth; I lifted weights. In other words, I didn't hesitate for a second when it came to doing whatever I could to stay young looking. (Definition of *young looking:* how I looked on my best day ten years prior to whatever *the present day* happened to be.)

So, I am not attempting to make facing the loss of my hair sound as if it was anything near a cakewalk. Not to mention the loss of both breasts. Or my ovaries. There were some serious tears shed, as well as some wee-small morning hours spent lying open-eyed on my pillow.

But, as keeping those physical parts of me didn't seem to be in my best interest at the time, we made surgery dates and chemo appointments. The process started, I mourned…and gave in to the rhythms of my prescribed healing dance card.

That's when something interesting occurred.

It was as if an invisible hand caught me by the collar and hoisted me up to cirrostratus level, allowing me a more encompassing view of my life. And, I seemed to hang there for several days, observing everyone and everything from this elevated vantage point.

Now, I don't know what your spiritual affiliation is (or if you even have one), but whatever your stance, I'd like to share with you a thought—a proverbial pearl in the poop—that was made abundantly clear to me during that time: A big part of learning to live fully is learning to let go.

Certainly, this type of letting go does not imply throwing in the towel on your looks or your life. Those sad choices never lead to a positive outcome. Rather, it's an invitation to act with wisdom when the time comes to release those things which we never held in permanent possession in the first place.

I really got it this time that if I expended all of my energy desperately trying to cling to an old status quo when life had insisted on serving me a new state of affairs, not only would that be an exercise in futility, but more importantly, I would be depriving myself of the priceless opportunity for growth.

Perhaps, to some, this might sound like a dubious cliché—a lame attempt to sugarcoat a sad situation because there's nothing else you can do about it, right?

I understand why you might feel that way. I used to, as well.

And, I'm not going to patronize you by telling you that "Cancer is such a gift," either. I find that statement to be way too small for its message. Besides, I like my gifts to be wrapped in satin ribbon—not surgical tubing.

No, I'm just saying that the way I see it now, having cancer gives us all a choice. We can fight it with our heads tucked against the relentless gale, pushing through it as best we can, eyes tightly shut until it's all over. (At least, we hope it's over as we find ourselves struggling daily to push away the nagging thought of its return.)

Or, we can fight it with an attitude of being open to learning all that we can from having this disease—physically, mentally, and spiritually—because we understand that there might be clues to a richer life buried deep within the experience.

That being said, I'd like to suggest you keep in mind the fact that you're not alone in facing change, though it sure might feel like it at this moment. *Everything* is constantly changing; it's just occurring at various speeds. You only have to stand beside one of the beautiful mountain streams so prevalent here in western North Carolina in January, and again in July, to see this fact beautifully evidenced.

The marvelous "existence parade" in which we're all participating, was obviously designed to keep moving, and trying to grab onto any part of the procession, is only going to create unnecessary pain. What are you gonna do? Jump a Shriner and wrestle him off his little scooter? Not only will you look pretty silly, but it will also cause you to miss the baton twirlers and marching band that's coming up next.

I can promise you that when we let go, while, at the same time, opening our minds and hearts—especially when we feel at our weakest or most fearful—we're tapping into our deepest strength of character. We are allowing the unlimited potential of healthy and joyous transformation.

Our souls grow deeper. Our paradigms, wider. Everything seems more precious. Problems become less worrisome.

Loss of hair...loss of breasts...not such a burden.

The following are lyrics to a song I wrote after I came through the other end of treatment. It's from the viewpoint of my own reflection in the mirror, if that image could talk to me:

YOU'RE STILL YOU

©2010 Lou Gideon

Take away your makeup
Take away your hair
Take away your eyebrows and lashes,
baby
You're still there

Take away your memory
Take a breast or two
(You say they're takin' what)
makes you a woman
Girl, that just ain't true

Somehow, you've got to get past
the notion
(Of thinking that) Right now
This illusion is "you"
Try once to see it from my point of view

(Time) took away my childhood
Where did that girl go?
(And though I can't) see her
She's still inside me, this I know

(So) take away the worry
Take away the fear
We are much more

Than the vision that's reflected here

Somehow, you've got to get
past the notion
(Of thinking that) Right now
This illusion is "you"
There's power in seeing from this
point of view

No matter what they have to do
to your bones or your body, baby
you're still you!

Still You
Beyond the heavens reaching light years
through the skies
Still You
Beyond reflections staring back into your
eyes
Still You
Beyond the limits here of earthly space
and time
Still You
A spark eternal in a cosmic grand design

I truly believe these words—no matter what my future holds. So, take a deep breath and smile, sister. We're all going to be just fine.

ACKNOWLEDGMENTS

I once heard it said that it takes an entire village to write a book, and now that this experience has taught me the undeniable truth in that little adage, there are a few special villagers I'd like to thank in particular:

My support team of friends and family who soldiered through the journey along with me by driving over, flying out, calling, laughing, and serving me an ongoing banquet of love, prayer, and buoyancy.

Callan and Janie, my sisters-in-strength warriors who never failed to be there for me day after day (and for all of Janie's tireless research); Marla M., for endless soul support and the many poignant insights we discovered together; Susan and Al, for flying out to smooth the way for my family during surgery, and for giving me a memorable hospital all-nighter of laughter and peace; Elizabeth, for supplying high vibes of the heart on the Carolina coastline; Robin, for her loving strength, and for the healing she brings from having the courage to say out loud what I'm thinking; Marla A., for late-night phone calls and a special pearl of great worth; Colleen, for wanting to give me her glorious hair if I chose to have a custom wig made, as well as all the gourmet nourishment she provided, mentally and physically; Joy, for her calming presence, uncanny perception, and basmati rice with raisins; Lark, for her elegant, constantly illuminating faith; Judith, for the priceless question she asked me three days after my diagnosis ("How are you going to turn this challenge into one of the best things that ever happened to you?"); Betsy, for her candid, uniquely Betsy-style humor, and for always being there when I needed her; Cissy, for providing Cissy-only magic; Lena, for her brand of "Love, Light, and Laughter;" Earleen for her optimism and generosity to so many of us survivor-thrivers; cousin Michael, for the consistent flow of love; my loving fellow Texan "sister" Pam, for her love, and for caring enough to rally the troops, if necessary; Chris and Doug, for being my anchors; Michael M., for his constant spiritual presence; Janis, for providing practical, loving input; Deborah, for her uplifting weekly cards; and Taylor, for donating to Locks of Love in my honor, for creating my one-of-a-kind art-pipe collection, and for just being Taylor.

As for the many other priceless friends who Facebooked, emailed, wrote to me, knitted prayer shawls, called, and sent flowers and thoughtful gifts: I want you to know that I'm incredibly grateful for every loving, supportive gesture—too many to count.

Thank you to Dr. Vladimir Lange, for his *Be a Survivor* series, and for his expert help and advice; Carol Reed for her time, care, and exuberance for getting the word out, as well as her great ideas; RF, for always believing in me, and for his graciousness in helping make this project happen; the good people at Proven Health Management; my caring team at Hope Women's Cancer Center, including the marvelous Dr. David Hetzel; and Dr. Donald R. Conway, for his artistry.

I'd especially like to thank the incomparable Micaela, for her unending patience, talent, recurring selfless efforts, and ongoing support. Also, a heartfelt thanks to Faiyaz and Gabrielle, my original "Remissionaries," for their patience and invaluable guidance maneuvering the mysterious land of publishing. I could not have completed this book without you!

Lastly, to my loving family: my sisters-in-law-to-be, Vicki and Melissa, for their love and prayers; Steve and Mel, my wonderful brother and sister-in-law, for their painstaking proofing and insights; Mom, for being my constant, uplifting angel in human form; Jazzy and Duhdley, for their particularly healing contribution of unconditional love and furry, tail-wagging support; and, most importantly, to the love of my life, Walt—for giving me the power to realize my dreams and the kind of love that makes accomplishing those dreams all the more worthwhile.

ABOUT THE AUTHOR

Lou Gideon was a writer and actress with over 35 years of experience in film, television, and theater, including multiple seasons on *Search for Tomorrow* and *The Secret World of Alex Mack*; along with guest spots on shows such as *Seinfeld*, *Night Court*, *Third Rock from the Sun*, and *Beverly Hills 90210*.

REDEDICATION

I am rededicating this book to my dear wife, Lou, who made her transition on February 3, 2014. She was blessed to always find the good in every situation—and was determined that, through her journey, she could help others find their strength, as well.

—*Walt Borchers*

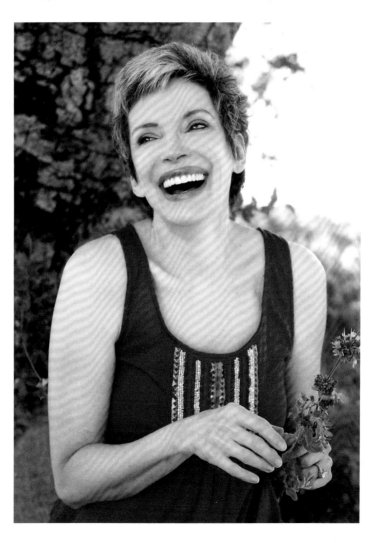